D1447615

More Advance Prais

Emergency Neurol

This is a
of comm   al prou.
likely to   ospital setting.
Each section is introduced by a clinical vignette which highlights the key points of presentation, physical findings and laboratory studies. These are well integrated in the discussion which reviews the differential diagnoses possible. Appropriate therapies are also reviewed. A list of suggested readings accompanies each vignette.

This book would be an excellent resource for residents and advanced practitioners. It helps focus neurological clinical reasoning. The author's clinical experience can be clearly seen in the reasoned discussion that follows each vignette. It was a pleasure to read this book and feel as if you had an experienced colleague at your side.

— *James A.D. Otis, MD, Department of Neurology, Boston University, Boston, MA*

Morris Levin, a superb clinician and educator, has done an excellent job in writing a text that is comprehensible and readable. Each of the thirty-two "bite size" chapters begin with a case which serves as the theme, Clinicians practicing in the "trenches" will find the format centered on the question "what do I do now"? to be particularly useful. This text should make its way to the shelf of all Internal Medicine hospitalists and general neurologists. Neurology residents will find the text to be an excellent resource particularly when on call.

— *David J. Capobianco, MD, Department of Neurology, Mayo Clinic, Jacksonville, FL*

What Do I Do Now?

SERIES CO-EDITORS-IN-CHIEF

Lawrence C. Newman, MD
Director of the Headache Institute
Department of Neurology
St. Luke's-Roosevelt Hospital Center
New York, NY

Morris Levin, MD
Professor of Neurology and Psychiatry
Geisel School of Medicine at Dartmouth
Hanover, NH

PREVIOUS VOLUMES IN THE SERIES

Headache and Facial Pain
Peripheral Nerve and Muscle Disease
Pediatric Neurology
Stroke
Epilepsy
Neurocritical Care
Neuro-Ophthalmology
Neuroimmunology
Pain
Neuroinfections

Emergency Neurology

Morris Levin, MD
Professor of Neurology and Psychiatry
Geisel School of Medicine at Dartmouth
Hanover, NH

OXFORD
UNIVERSITY PRESS

Oxford University Press is a department of the University of Oxford.
It furthers the University's objective of excellence in research, scholarship,
and education by publishing worldwide.

Oxford   New York
Auckland   Cape Town   Dar es Salaam   Hong Kong   Karachi
Kuala Lumpur   Madrid   Melbourne   Mexico City   Nairobi
New Delhi   Shanghai   Taipei   Toronto

With offices in
Argentina   Austria   Brazil   Chile   Czech Republic   France   Greece
Guatemala   Hungary   Italy   Japan   Poland   Portugal   Singapore
South Korea   Switzerland   Thailand   Turkey   Ukraine   Vietnam

Oxford is a registered trademark of Oxford University Press in the UK and
certain other countries.

Published in the United States of America by
Oxford University Press
198 Madison Avenue, New York, NY 10016

Library of Congress Cataloging-in-Publication Data
Levin, Morris, 1955–
Emergency neurology / Morris Levin.
    p. ; cm.—(What do I do now?)
Includes bibliographical references and index.
ISBN 978–0–19–986285–6 (pbk. : alk. paper)
I. Title.   II. Series: What do I do now?
[DNLM: 1. Central Nervous System Diseases—Case Reports.   2. Emergencies—Case Reports.
3. Adult.   4. Child. WL 301]

616.8025—dc23
2012041107

Printed in the United States of America
on acid-free paper

This book is dedicated to my beautiful and brilliant wife, Karen, who knew, vaguely, what I was doing in my office late at night these last weeks, and was tolerant of this latest in a long line of projects of mine.

—ML

Preface

Neurologists are regular consultants either in person or by phone for emergency departments the world over. Case types range from clear neurological syndromes to complex or "overlap" presentations with psychiatric, cardiologic, pulmonary, and other features. Some of the most perplexing cases seen in emergency or urgent settings land in the territory of neurologists. Sometimes, this is because all of the obvious etiological agents have been ruled out and perhaps, diagnostically, something neurological or neuropsychiatric is at play. Other emergent neurological consultations are primarily treatment issues, for example, those patients who present with a stroke syndrome not completely fitting into a protocol category. And sometimes a challenging ethical dilemma is encountered revolving around a patient's awareness or capacity for decision-making.

Many of these consultations arise after the ED staff becomes stumped, and neurologists, too, may be stymied, asking themselves "What do I do now?" Using standard textbooks or reviewing literature may often be unproductive or, at the very least, too slow for the inherent need for speed in the emergency setting. Tracking down the correct subspecialist neurologist can be difficult. Hence, there is a need for a quick reference tool that could serve as a resource for some of these difficult emergency neurology conundrums.

I, with the help of some of my neurological colleagues, have identified 32 commonly encountered emergency neurological consultation situations that are often rather perplexing. I have, in keeping with the format of the "What do I do now" series, presented these in the form of a brief case vignette, followed by a discussion of options. I have simulated the "curbside consultation" in which the key questions in each are addressed, much as a consultant would do over the phone or in the hallway. And as in real life, correct answers may be negotiable. The cases in this volume are divided into four sections that cover the typical ground for emergency neurological consultation: (1) Diagnostic Questions (adult); (2) Treatment Considerations (adult); (3) Ethical, Neuropsychiatric, and Legal issues; and (4) Pediatric issues. Recommendations discussed are based on the most current evidence available, but should not be taken as bona fide guidelines.

Diagnostic thinking is presented hierarchically with important/common diagnoses handled first. Treatment decision-making is weighted by evidence and safety. A list of key clinical points appears at the end of each case discussion. Also in keeping with the format of this series, extensive referencing is not attempted, but, at the end of each case discussion, there is a list of suggested articles or chapters for those interested in doing further reading on the subject. Tables are provided for quick reference in some chapters.

This book is designed as a resource for clinicians at all levels of training in all fields of medicine, who treat patients with urgent, emergent, and/ or critical care neurological syndromes. It uses a novel approach akin to case-based learning and emphasizes the creative intellectual process we all relish. It can be used as a handy reference for common troublesome questions, but can also serve as a rehearsal tool to prepare the busy consultant for a number of eventualities. Finally, it can be used as a self-assessment tool by pausing after reading each case to formulate a diagnosis and plan; then reading on to see suggestions in the text. I hope it serves the purpose of making some difficult presentations in emergency neurology more manageable to the clinician. Thanks for reading.

Morris Levin, MD
Hanover, New Hampshire

Contents

PART II   THERAPEUTIC DILEMMAS IN ADULT PATIENTS

Abbreviations

AP	Anterior-posterior
BID	Twice a day
BP	Blood pressure
CBC	Complete blood count
CK	Creatine kinase
COPD	Chronic obstructive pulmonary disease
CSF	Cerebrospinal fluid
CT	Computerized tomography
CTA	Computerized tomography angiography
ECG	Electrocardiogram
EEG	Electroencephalogram
ED	Emergency department
ER	Emergency room
ESR	Erythrocyte sedimentation rate
HEENT	Head, ears, eyes, nose and throat
IM	Intramuscular
IV	Intravenous
LP	Lumbar puncture
MRI	Magnetic resonance imaging
MRA	Magnetic resonance angiography
MS	Multiple sclerosis
NSAID	Non-steroidal anti-inflammatory drug
OTC	Over the counter
PCR	Polymerase chain reaction test
QHS	At bedtime
RBC	Red blood cell
RF	Rheumatoid factor
TIA	Transient ischemic attack
WBC	White blood cell
oC	Degrees Centigrade
oF	Degrees Fahrenheit

PART I

Diagnostic Dilemmas in Adult Patients

Coma with Fever

A 26-year-old man was found unresponsive in his apartment by a neighbor. He was brought to the emergency department (ED) by ambulance. No history is known other than he lives alone and works as a cook at a local restaurant. He has a temperature of 102° F, blood pressure of 128/60, and pulse rate of 100. Breathing is regular and deep at a rate of 14. His neck is slightly stiff in flexion/extension but not in rotation. Head, ears, eyes, nose, and throat (HEENT) are normal in appearance. Lungs are clear and cardiac auscultation reveals only a soft midsystolic murmur. Abdomen is not tender. There is no rash or other skin abnormality. He does not arouse to any stimuli. Pupils are 4 mm in diameter and react to light equally. Corneal reflexes are intact. Oculocephalic reflex is normal. He moves his extremities sluggishly in response to painful stimulation with some suggestion of decreased power in his left leg. Electrocardiogram (ECG) is normal. Chest x-ray has not been done yet. Blood count reveals white blood cell count of 14,000, red blood cell count of 39,000, and electrolytes are normal. He has been given glucose and naloxone with no response. You are consulted to come and do a lumbar puncture (LP) because the ED staff has tried and failed.

What do you do now?

This seriously ill, perhaps even fatally ill, patient requires quick diagnostic and treatment decision-making. The questions you began considering, even on the way to the ED, of course, were whether further delay in obtaining cerebrospinal fluid (CSF) is allowable and whether a dangerous mass lesion might be hiding intracranially. The two are connected, of course, because puncturing the dura in a patient with increased intracranial pressure, particularly if asymmetrical as in the case of a temporal mass lesion, could lead to transtentorial herniation, clinical worsening, and even death. So, a computed tomography (CT) image of the head is warranted immediately if a LP is needed (which is certainly the case here). But there has already been delay, and waiting for the CT will add further delay. So, the first step is obvious once you realize that your primary job is to lessen the danger here – starting broad-coverage antimicrobial therapy immediately, in order to at least begin to treat what might be a life-threatening meningitis or encephalitis. Once this is started, proceeding to CT in a brisk fashion, followed by LP will be possible. Blood cultures can be quite helpful and can easily be sent before antibiotics are started.

Interestingly, what we were taught in medical school about the nature of meningismus is correct: stiffness in flexion-extension is indicative of meningeal irritation; stiffness in rotation is not. Therefore this patient clearly has meningismus. In this age group, meningitis can be caused by a number of organisms, and surprisingly, the relative probability of various organisms has changed somewhat over the past few years, probably as a result of the H. influenza and S. pneumoniae vaccines. For example, gram-negative bacteria and Staphylococci have overtaken Strep in some areas as the most common cause. And despite advances in antibiotic choices and early diagnosis, approximately 10%–20% of adults with meningitis will die from it and another similar percentage will experience significant sequelae from it. Initial choices in antibiotic therapy should still consist of ceftriaxone (2 gm IV q 12 hours) and vancomycin (1.5 gm IV q 12 hours) with the possible addition of ampicillin if Listeria is suspected (e.g., in elderly or immune-compromised patients). There is growing resistance to even these antibiotics, however, which unfortunately makes culture results even more important. Nosocomial causes of meningitis, as well as suspected meningitis after penetrating head injury, lead to different etiological considerations, which are not at issue with this case.

Cerebrospinal fluid should be Gram-stained and cultured. In this particular case, if this patient does have bacterial meningitis, there may be a problem in identifying the causative organism, since antibiotics were begun before CSF was obtained. Fortunately, for most bacterial causes of meningitis, cultures will be positive even after antibiotics are started. This is less true for Neisseria, but for all bacterial causes, Gram-stain data will be abnormal for many hours, and neutrophil-prominent pleocytosis will persist as well. Low glucose and high protein will likewise be present for some time after treatment is begun (see Table 1.1 for typical CSF patterns in different meningitides). If lab evaluation is equivocal, polymerase chain reaction (PCR) testing for common causal organisms may be obtained, although this is not yet commonly available and sensitivity may not be ideal. Herpes simplex virus PCR should always be done if there is any chance of viral encephalitis. This patient should also be investigated for other infectious diseases and head magnetic resonance imaging (MRI), magnetic resonance angiogram (MRA) (to assess for possible arteritis), and magnetic resonance venogram (MRV) (to exclude cerebral venous thrombosis) should be done if the patient does not improve.

The addition of corticosteroids acutely in the management of strongly suspected bacterial meningitis is generally done at high dose as soon as possible, despite some conflicting evidence of efficacy. A common approach is to use dexamethasone 10 mg every 6 hours intravenously (IV) for several days when Gram stain is positive and CSF pleocytosis is present.

TABLE 1.1 **CSF Patterns in Meningitis of Various Etiologies**

	White blood cells	Protein	Glucose
Bacterial meningitis	++neutrophils	high	low
TB, Fungal meningitis	++lymphocytes	high	low
Carcinomatous, sarcoid meningitis	++lymphocytes	high	low
Viral, parasitic meningitis	++lymphocytes	high	normal
Viral encephalitis	+lymphocytes	high or normal	normal
Partially treated bacterial meningitis	+lymphocytes	high	normal

Patients with suspected bacterial meningitis should be placed in respiratory isolation for the first day of treatment if possible until the organism is identified. Patients with meningococcal meningitis should remain on droplet precautions for at least 24 hours after antibiotics are begun, although specific guidelines vary. Pneumococcal and viral causes do not require isolation. Meningococcal meningitis contacts should be treated prophylactically once the organism is identified depending upon local policy.

KEY POINTS TO REMEMBER

- Bacterial meningitis must be treated with a broad-coverage antibiotic regimen as soon as possible to prevent morbidity and mortality even if this means treating prior to obtaining CSF.
- Bacterial cultures can be helpful in choosing antibiotic therapy even if antibiotics have been started.
- CSF Gram-stain and white-blood-cell results remain abnormal for many hours following the initiation of antibiotics.
- Corticosteroids are probably effective in reducing morbidity in bacterial meningitis and pose little risk in terms of adverse effects.

Further Reading

Durand ML, Calderwood SB, Weber DJ, et al. Acute bacterial meningitis in adults–a review of 493 episodes. *N Engl J Med.* 1993;328:21-28.

Hasbun R, Abrahams J, Jekel J, et al. Computed tomography of the head before lumbar puncture in adults with suspected meningitis. *N Engl J Med.* 2001;345(24):1727-1733.

Tunkel AR, Hartman BJ, Kaplan SL, et al. Practice guidelines for the management of bacterial meningitis. *Clin Infect Dis.* 2004;39(9):1267-1284.

Agitated Delirium

A 31-year-old man was brought to the ED by the police in a confused and agitated state. He needed to be restrained by the staff in order to obtain blood for testing. He had been resistant to oral thermometer, but after sedation with lorazepam rectal temperature was obtained and was 99°F. Blood pressure (BP) is 180/88 and pulse rate is 110. A lumbar puncture was not deemed safe and the CT tech has refused to accept the patient as he is too combative, despite a second dose of lorazepam intravenously. No medical history is available as he has never been in your hospital before. On exam, the patient is unkempt, but no signs of trauma are noted. Respirations seem regular at a rate of 20. HEENT are normal, neck is supple, and lungs are clear. Abdomen seems a bit tense but palpation did not seem to be painful. The patient is awake, but does not respond to verbal communication other than to moan loudly. Pupils are dilated (5 mm bilaterally) but reactive. Eye movements seem intact and conjugate. He moves all extremities vigorously. Reflexes are brisk diffusely. Plantar reflexes are equivocal. Electrolytes, BUN, and creatinine are normal. Chest x-ray has not been done. Urine obtained via catheterization revealed normal urinalysis and routine drug screen was positive only for marijuana.

What do you do now?

This not uncommon presentation of agitated confusion, or delirium, is daunting. Serious life-threatening illness may underlie it, which must be discovered as soon as possible. And perhaps even more urgently, this patient must be sedated to at least some extent to prevent injury to himself and others. Haloperidol intramuscularly is a good default approach in the 2–10 mg dose range. It is relatively nontoxic, although it does require hepatic action and in patients with liver disease caution must be exercised. It does not have respiratory depressing actions, unlike benzodiazepines, and its duration of action is at least 3–4 hours.

Once the patient has been sedated, and this should take no more than a few minutes, a neurological exam can be attempted. Respiratory drive must be assessed as it is crucial to predict whether intubation and ventilatory assistance will soon be required. One of the most important assessments is to gauge whether consciousness is waning as this is a significant predictive factor. Mental status evaluation will, of course, be challenging, but it will be important to see if language is intact because aphasia can mimic confusion. Cranial nerve dysfunction can suggest brainstem involvement or a process in the subarachnoid space such as meningeal infection or inflammation. Motor exam can provide clues as to hemispheric localization. Sensation evaluation is cursory at best, and essentially consists of assessing the patient's response to sensory stimulation. Reflexes can help, although symmetry is the only real parameter that is trustworthy. Coordination can be estimated. Gait in cases like this is virtually impossible to assess. General exam, with a focus on signs of head trauma, liver or renal stigmata, cardiovascular details, and skin lesions/rashes, may provide clues in these cases. Pupillary changes in delirium can also provide clues. Anticholinergics such as atropine, scopolamine, and medications with anticholinergic properties, such as tricyclic antidepressants, cause mydriasis by antagonizing muscarinic receptors in the iris. Psychedelics such as LSD, psilocybin, and mescaline also produce mydriasis, but by agonizing central serotonin (5-HT2A) receptors. Drugs that increase serotonin activity in general, such as the selective serotonin reuptake inhibitor (SSRI) antidepressants, can do the same thing. Dissociative drugs such as phencyclicine (PCP) and ketamine antagonize NMDA glutamate receptors, which also can lead to mydriasis. Agents with adrenergic boosting properties including cocaine and amphetamines including Ecstasy (MDMA) and "crystal meth" (methamphetamine) can also produce mydriasis. Opioids do not cause mydriasis, rather they lead to miosis (as does ethanol), but withdrawal from opioids can indeed lead to papillary dilation. Marijuana generally causes injection of the sclera but may lead to some pupilodilation.

The differential diagnosis for agitated delirium is large, and while some possibilities have been excluded here with basic lab testing many remain. Vascular disorders that may cause delirium include acute stroke, subarachnoid hemorrhage, and intracerebral hemorrhage. To rule these out, CT of the head is necessary, hence the urgent need for sedation. Infectious causes including encephalitis require CSF evaluation, which will also complete the workup for subarachnoid hemorrhage. Herpes encephalitis is always a possibility as are seasonal encephalitides like West Nile virus, which can present with a meningoencephalitic picture—fever, stiff neck, and confusion. Glucose, protein, Veneral Disease Research Laboratory test (VDRL), cultures, stains (Gram, acid fast, India ink), and herpes PCR are all ordered. If the patient is febrile, blood cultures are also ordered and, in cases like this, might be worthwhile even if the patient is afebrile. Serum VDRL, human immunodefiency virus (HIV), Lyme, and toxoplasmosis titers are all considerations. CSF will also help assess the presence of cerebral vasculitis, where protein elevation is nearly universal. Head trauma, which may have occurred despite the absence of superficial signs of recent injury, can lead to delirium due to subdural hematoma or intracranial contusion. A plethora of metabolic factors can lead to delirium including hepatic encephalopathy, uremia, hyponatremia, hypoxia, hypercapnia, hypo or hyperglycemia, porphyria, thyrotoxicosis, Cushing's disease, Addison's disease, and Wernicke's encephalopathy. So, in addition to basic metabolic panel and complete blood count (CBC), liver enzymes and thyroid screen should at least be done.

Drug/alcohol intoxication or withdrawal in some settings is highly likely in cases presenting with delirium. Possibilities are numerous and include accidental or intentional overdose of prescription medications, such as sedatives, antidepressants, antipsychotics, opioids, antiepileptics, lithium, antihistamines, dopaminergics, anticholinergics, and stimulants. Illicit-drug-induced confusional states are common and include a number of new cannabinoids and stimulants sold legally in many states (e.g., "bath salts," "inhaled incense"), in addition to cocaine, opioids, amphetamines, barbiturates, and psychedelics. Typically, hospital urine drug testing includes the following drugs:

- Alcohol (ethanol)
- Amphetamines
- Analgesics (acetaminophen and anti-inflammatory drugs)
- Antidepressants
- Barbiturates
- Benzodiazepines
- Cocaine
- Flunitrazepam (Rohypnol)
- Marijuana
- Opioids
- Phencyclidine (PCP)
- Phenothiazines and other neuroleptic drugs

When drug screen is negative, most hospital labs have more inclusive drug screen panels that can be done or sent out.

Rare paraneoplastic syndromes include limbic encephalitis (most commonly seen in small-cell lung cancer, sometimes with anti-Hu antibodies) and anti-NMDA receptor encephalitis (often in gonadal cancer). Epilepsy can be the cause of confusional states, even agitated delirium, in several ways. Nonconvulsive status epilepticus generally does not produce agitation but rather an abulic, withdrawn presentation; it remains, however, a possibility that is difficult to rule out without an electroencephalogram (EEG). Some physicians will try IV lorazepam in an attempt to stop the epileptic activity, but this may only serve to sedate the patient. EEG can also help to identify some metabolic causes of delirium, including hepatic encephalopathy with the appearance of triphasic waves. Postictal confusion can present with agitation as well. The time course is usually diagnostic with resolution, or even sleep, occurring after some time. Finally, antiepileptic medication effect can be causal, for example, due to gradual elevation of blood levels of one or more antiepileptic drugs (AEDs) in a patient with difficulty controlling seizures who is being tapered upward on medications.

Initial treatment, even before CT and LP are attempted should always include naloxone (Narcan) 1–2 amps IV or intramuscularly (IM) every

5 minutes to prevent respiratory depression, which could be imminent after opioid overdose. Conversely, flumazenil .2 mg (2 ml) over 30 seconds can be administered if the cause of the confusional state is known to be due to benzodiazepine overdose, but should NOT be given when this is not clear as it can lead to seizures, even status epilepticus, in patients with epilepsy. Glucose is always given even before labs are sent, and presumably this was done in this case even before you were called.

If Wernicke's encephalopathy is possible, thiamine 100 mg IM should be routinely given.

So, this patient needs to be sedated quickly, have some initial treatment given, have a brain CT done as soon as possible, and possibly LP and EEG if the diagnosis is not made quickly. Serial neurological exams should be done frequently to assess for deterioration. There should be low threshold for intubation if the patient seems to be dropping his respiratory drive. More extensive drug screening should be considered, and a quest to obtain more medical history should be undertaken.

KEY POINTS TO REMEMBER

- Agitated confusion poses risks both to the patient and the medical team.
- Sedation of delirious patients should be given as soon as it is deemed necessary; the choice should be made between parenteral benzodiazepine and neuroleptic medication.
- Initial treatment in delirium should include glucose, naloxone, and thiamine.
- In confused patients where diagnosis is not clear, head CT is essential.
- When meningitis or encephalitis is possible, LP should not be delayed.
- Intoxication with prescription, over-the-counter, and illicit drugs should ALWAYS be suspected in the delirious patient.

Further Reading

Mayo-Smith MF, Beecher LH, Fischer TL, et al. Management of alcohol withdrawal delirium. An evidence-based practice guideline. *Arch Intern Med.* 2004;164(13):1405-1412.
Rossi J, Swan MC, Isaacs ED. The violent or agitated patient. *Emerg Med Clin North Am.* 2010;28:235-256.

3 Post Carotid Endarterectomy Neurological Deficit

A 68-year-old man who presented 6 days ago with transient language difficulty, was found to have high-grade left-internal carotid stenosis, and underwent left-carotid endarterectomy at another hospital 3 days ago. Today he awoke with numbness in his right arm, which has persisted all morning. His wife called 911 and he arrived at your ED by ambulance. Vital signs are normal, HEENT are normal, lungs are clear, and cardiac exam is normal. Neck is supple and the endarterectomy incision is healing well. However, there is a bruit over this carotid. On neurological exam, mental state, cranial nerves, strength, and coordination are all intact, but there does seem to be numbness over the entire right arm. CT scan is normal.

What do you do now?

V irtually every clinician treating adults knows that carotid endarterectomy has been proven effective for prophylactic treatment of symptomatic carotid stenosis. Few, however, have seen complications and feel comfortable dealing with them. All of the usual potential postsurgical adverse consequences can occur in these patients. Wound dehiscence and infection are very rare. The most common adverse sequelae include myocardial infection, transient ischemic attack (TIA), stroke, hyperperfusion syndrome, neck region nerve injury, and parotitis. Stroke in the perioperative period can result from a number of contributing causes including platelet aggregation and thrombosis formation, plaque emboli, carotid dissection, and relatively low cerebral arterial perfusion pressure. The etiology of TIA or stroke must be assessed as well as possible in order to choose the appropriate treatment.

After symptoms that could relate to carotid disease develop, the first step, and one that must be done quickly, is to get a reliable visualization of the carotid artery. This is best done via intra-arterial angiography to detect the flow-limiting dissection or thrombosis, but CT angiography is often quicker and nearly as useful. If either dissection or thrombosis is found, heparinization has traditionally been the treatment of choice. Prior to this, most would agree that the patient should undergo CT scanning of the head to rule out intracranial hemorrhage. Some surgeons favor surgical re-exploration if complications happen very early, but more recently, percutaneous carotid angioplasty with direct stenting is felt to be potentially very useful for postoperative carotid occlusion. Many case reports document remission of neurological symptoms if stenting is done quickly, and a case series comparing stenting to surgical re-exploration published in 2001 attests to this.

Intra-arterial thrombolytic therapy, in select cases, may be another treatment option in patients with a postoperative thrombotic stroke suggested by arteriography. The rationale for the administration of tissue-type plasminogen activator (tPA) for these patients is based upon its proven success in acute stroke, but there is no clear evidence to support this yet.

An important syndrome to exclude is the hyperperfusion syndrome (HPS) which can produce three characteristic conditions: (1) persistent headache, (2) intracerebral hemorrhage, or (3) focal seizures. This last can involve significant post-seizure ("Todds") paralysis, which can be misleading. Hyperperfusion syndrome (HPS) tends to occur 3–10 days following endarterectomy. The etiology of the HPS is thought to be due to some degree of cerebral autoregulation breakdown due to the large change in flow. It might be difficult to differentiate hyperperfusion consequences from perior postoperative stroke. Head CT and MRI with T2 or Fluid-attenuated Inversion- Recovery (FLAIR) sequences typically show cerebral edema with or without intracerebral hemorrhage. Transcranial Doppler testing can reveal cerebral hyperperfusion, and single-photon emission computed tomography (SPECT) can also be useful. Strict control of systemic hypertension is the best way to treat HPS, and this may require labetalol or nitroprusside.

Since cranial nerves can be damaged during operative procedure, this cause of neurological deficits must also be excluded if cranial nerve symptoms and signs tend to predominate (unlike the case above). Nerves at risk include (1) vagus nerve, which if damaged can lead to vocal cord paralysis; (2) portions of the facial nerve, leading to an asymmetric smile; (3) branches of the trigeminal nerve, resulting in facial sensory loss; and finally (4) the hypoglossal nerve, which may result in tongue deviation to the side of injury. Nerve damage is generally due to traction, but transection is also possible. The most reliable predictor of cranial nerve injury during endarterectomy is surgery duration, with a very low likelihood of cranial nerve damage in patients whose time in the operating room was less than 2 hours.

KEY POINTS TO REMEMBER

- Carotid endarterectomy is generally safe, but postoperative complications include stroke and hyperperfusion syndrome.
- In endarterectomy patients who develop focal deficits in the perioperative period, immediate CT of the head is recommended to exclude hemorrhage.
- Vascular imaging is essential to determine the presence of thrombosis or dissection of the carotid artery.
- Anticoagulation is the standard treatment for post-endarterectomy thrombosis or dissection, but intra-arterial thrombolysis and stenting are alternatives that are being studied.
- Assessment of cranial arterial blood flow is important in determining the presence of the hyperperfusion syndrome.
- Management of arterial blood pressure is crucial if hyperperfusion syndrome is suspected.

Further Reading

Adhiyaman V, Alexander S. Cerebral hyperperfusion syndrome following carotid endarterectomy. *Q J Med.* 2007;100:239-244.

Anzuini A, Briguori C, Roubin G, Rosanio S, et al. Emergency stenting to treat neurological complications occurring after carotid endarterectomy. *J Am Coll Cardiol.* 2001;37:2074-2079.

Flanigan DP, Flanigan ME, Dorne AL, et al. Long-term results of 442 consecutive, standardized carotid endarterectomy procedures in standard-risk and high-risk patients. *J Vasc Surg.* 2007;46:876-882.

Persistent Migraine Aura

A 48-year-old woman with a several-year history of migraine with aura describes to the ED physician the onset of one of her typical migraines the day before. She also describes her typical visual aura symptoms, including blurred vision, scintillations, and apparent loss of vision in the "left eye." She states that the headache abated with oral sumatriptan but the visual symptoms have not. The longest an aura has lasted in the past is approximately 60 minutes. She also feels anxious and a bit confused, but on mental status testing she seems intact. Cranial-nerve exam is normal except for visual acuity, which is decreased bilaterally. Funduscopy is normal and the ophthalmology consultant has seen the patient and has excluded ocular disease. There does seem to be a left visual field deficit involving both upper and lower visual quadrants. Motor exam is normal with intact symmetrical reflexes. Sensory exam is generally normal, but there may be some diminution to light touch and vibration in the right arm and trunk. Coordination is intact, but gait seems limited by vision. CT of the head with and without contrast is normal, as is basic hematology and chemistry blood testing.

What do you do now?

This patient has relatively typical migraine aura symptoms (visual and sensory), but of atypical duration. The International Classification of Headache Disorders, 2nd edition, published by the International Headache Society in 2004, defines Persistent migraine aura as lasting more than 1 week without radiographic evidence of infarction. A second entity, Migrainous infarction, is defined as "one or more aura symptoms [which] persists for > 60 minutes" and where "Neuroimaging demonstrates ischaemic infarction in a relevant area." (See Tables 4.1 and 4.2.) Our patient fits neither definition. An important deciding diagnostic test is MRI with diffusion-weighted imaging (DWI). If this is positive, it is very possible migrainous stroke has occurred. Migraine itself is a mild risk factor for stroke, particularly in certain populations, most notably young women. This is primarily limited to patients who experience migraine auras, although migraine without aura also carries an overall mildly increased risk of stroke. An unanswered question is whether longer than average duration of aura symptoms is a more significant risk. Also unanswered, and of great interest, is the question of stroke pathophysiology in migraine. Presumably this is related either to some migraine induced circulatory compromise or hypermetabolic "exhaustion" of normal perfusion, leading to relative ischemia to one or more brain regions.

If the MRI is negative, however, there are still two important imperatives: (1) to continue to investigate possible causes of ischemia or other possible causes of prolonged aura-like symptoms and (2) to attempt to curtail the aura. A number of conditions may mimic prolonged auras, including occipital lobe epilepsy, vertebrobasilar transient ischemic attacks, cerebral venous thrombosis, reversible cerebral vasoconstriction syndrome (RCVS),

TABLE 4.1 **International Classification of Headache Disorders, 2nd edition: Persistent aura without infarction**

Description:
Aura symptoms persist for more than 1 week without radiographic evidence of infarction.
Diagnostic criteria:
   A. The present attack in a patient with Migraine with aura is typical of previous attacks except that one or more aura symptoms persists for > 1 week
   B. Not attributed to another disorder

Description:
One or more migrainous aura symptoms associated with an ischaemic brain lesion in appropriate territory demonstrated by neuroimaging.
Diagnostic criteria:
  A. The present attack in a patient with 1.2 Migraine with aura is typical of previous attacks except that one or more aura symptoms persists for > 60 minutes
  B. Neuroimaging demonstrates ischaemic infarction in a relevant area
  C. Not attributed to another disorder

carotid or vertebral artery dissection, cerebral vasculitis, and hematological diseases causing "sludging." Mitochondrial encephalopathy, lactic acidosis, and stroke-like episodes (MELAS) syndrome and cerebral autosomal dominant arteriopathy with subcortical infarcts and leukoencephalopathy (CADASIL) are two other possibilities that MRI should exclude. CT angiography (CTA) may be necessary in cases of prolonged aura to exclude vasculitis and RCVS. Imaging of the neck vessels with CTA or MRA may also be appropriate. EEG is very useful not only in excluding ongoing epileptic activity, but also in corroborating neurophysiological alterations in the cortex corresponding to the patient's symptoms. In the patient above, one would expect to see slowing or some altered electrophysiological activity in right posterior derivations.

There are no clear treatment guidelines for patients suffering from prolonged migraine auras. Historically, despite a lack of evidence of real benefit, inhalation therapy with 10% carbon dioxide and 90% oxygen, amyl nitrate or isoproterenol, and sublingual nifedipine have been used, based on the theory that migrainous auras were the result of prolonged vasoconstriction. In addition, recent studies of patients with prolonged migraine aura have found areas of cortical hypoperfusion corresponding to the region of aura symptoms. However, it seems that this is the result of a decreased metabolic demand rather than an ischemic mechanism, so presumably there is ongoing cortical spreading depression in these patients, which might respond to a different therapeutic approach. Hence, a number of agents have been tried including magnesium sulfate, prochlorperazine, divalproex, acetazolamide, verapamil, flunarizine, lamotrigine, gabapentin, and memantine.

Intravenous magnesium sulfate is probably a good place to start due to its relative safety, followed by intravenous divalproex.

So, in summary, with prolonged migraine aura it is imperative to look further for evidence of cerebral ischemia and other causes of focal neurological deficits, which can then be explored and managed. If there is no stroke on MRI DWI images, persistent aura is the most likely diagnosis, although this is not considered conclusive until the aura symptoms have lasted more than 1 week, with imaging remaining normal. There are several options, but no clear guidelines, for treating the aura in hopes of curtailing it. Finally, while little is known about the etiology of risk factors, sequelae, and best treatment for patients with prolonged migraine aura, the presentation is worrisome and migraine preventive measures should be instituted.

KEY POINTS TO REMEMBER

- Migraine auras typically develop over 5–20 minutes and resolve within 1 hour or less.
- When aura lasts beyond 1 hour, investigation into other possible causes of focal neurological deficits should be considered.
- MRI with DWI should be abnormal in migrainous infarction, and MR or CT imaging along with EEG can generally rule out other pathological causes.
- Treatments that have helped some patients to halt prolonged auras include magnesium sulfate, divalproex, oxygen, and verapimil.

Further Reading

Headache Classification Committee of the International Headache Society. International Classification of Headache Disorders. 2nd ed. *Cephalalgia.* 2004;24:S9-S160.

Kurth T, Diener H. Current views of the risk of stroke for migraine with and migraine without aura. *Curr Pain Headache Rep.* 2006;10:214-220.

Rothrock JF, Walicke P, Swenson MR, Lyden PD, Logan WR. Migrainous stroke. *Arch Neurol.* 1988;45:63-67.

Rozen TD. Aborting a prolonged migrainous aura with intravenous prochlorperazine and magnesium sulfate. *Headache* 2003;43:901-903.

Stefano Viola S, Viola P, Litterio P, Buongarzone MP, Fiorelli L. "Prolonged" migraine aura: New information on underlying mechanisms. *Translational Neuroscience.* 2011;2:101-105.

5 Contraindication to Lumbar Puncture

A 32-year-old man with idiopathic thrombocytopenic purpura (ITP) is brought to the ED due to confusion. He complains of a moderate headache but is otherwise comfortable. He is awake with reasonably intact language but is disoriented to date, unable to count backwards, and does not remember recent events. His vital signs are normal save for a temperature of 100°F. Neck is supple, lungs are clear, cardiac exam is normal, abdomen is soft and non-tender, and there are no skin changes. His platelet count is 40,000, RBC count is 4.8 million, and WBC count is 10,000. CT scan of the head is reported as normal. While the ED physician is pondering the next steps, the patient is observed to have a brief generalized seizure, after which he is somnolent but still nonfocal in exam. After coming to see the patient, who now, 15 minutes after the convulsive seizure, is back at his original baseline, you observe that his neck may not be completely supple in the anterior-posterior direction, and that there is a right-sided Babinski reflex.

What do you do now?

In general, the main indications for LP are (1) to rule out meningitis and encephalitis; (2) to diagnose subarachnoid hemorrhage; and (3) to assess opening pressure. The main contraindications are (1) markedly increased intracranial pressure (for fear of causing transtentorial or cerebellar herniations); (2) infection at the site of lumbar puncture; and (3) bleeding diathesis (for fear of inducing epidural or intrathecal hemorrhage). Here, there is strong suspicion for encephalitis or meningoencephalitis, where speedy diagnosis is truly crucial, but there is also an equally important contraindication. Because early institution of antimicrobial medication has been shown to improve patient outcomes in meningitis and encephalitis significantly, broad-coverage antibiotics (ceftriaxone and vancomycin) along with acyclovir should be started immediately. The decision about adding corticosteroids can be put on hold temporarily.

But before a LP can be performed something needs to be done about the thrombocytopenia. Right? Not necessarily. There have been a number of studies looking at risks of spinal hematomata in patients with thrombocytopenia from various causes, particularly ITP. In patients with platelet counts above 40,000/cc the risk seems to be small. To decrease the risk in patients with lower counts, many hematologists recommend transfusing platelets to get the count above 50,000/cc. The transfusion should be done immediately prior to LP. There may be a time delay arranging for transfusion, and administering it, hence the importance of beginning antibiotics beforehand in patients like this one.

As for other causes of bleeding diathesis, consultation with a hematologist can be enormously helpful. For patients receiving pharmacological anticoagulation, the following guidelines should be followed prior to performing lumbar puncture: Warfarin should be discontinued; vitamin K should be injected or fresh-frozen plasma (FFP) transfused, or both, with the goal of producing an international normalized ratio (INR) below 1.2; heparin should be discontinued and partial thromboplastin time (PTT) normalized with protamine. The dosage for heparin reversal is 1 mg protamine sulfate IV for every 100 IU of active heparin. It was initially derived from fish, and while it is now synthetically produced via a recombinant DNA process, patients who are allergic to fish can develop a histamine reaction with hypotension, bronchoconstriction, and skin reaction. Diabetes and fast infusion of protamine also seem to increase the risk of an adverse reaction.

Reinstatement of intravenous heparin should not be done for at least 1 hour after the procedure. Low molecular weight heparin (LMWH) has a longer half-life than heparin and is not reversible with protamine, so, it is prudent to wait 12–24 hours before LP unless FFP is given. Close neurologic monitoring (mental state, cranial nerve function, motor function, and sensory function) should be performed for at least 24 hours post-LP to ensure prompt recognition and treatment of a spinal hematoma. There do not seem to be significant concerns regarding LP in patients on NSAIDs or the need for post-LP monitoring.

Interestingly, in patients with normal coagulation, there is still a finite risk of bleeding complications, probably less than 1% but not negligible. Certainly some of these patients may have underlying coagulation dysfunction that only comes to light later. But this suggests that perhaps prior to LP, bleeding parameters should be done, which is not always common practice. Other complications of lumbar puncture must also be kept in mind following the procedure, including post-dural puncture headache, cranial neuropathies, nerve root irritation, low back pain, and infections, including nosocomial meningitis.

So, this patient is probably safe to undergo LP, even without correction of platelet count. The 40,000 platelet count is borderline, however, and transfusion of platelets could be done. Speed is important but not crucial as antibiotic coverage has already been expedited. Antiepileptic medication should be loaded to prevent further epileptic seizures, which could be dangerous during LP.

KEY POINTS TO REMEMBER

- Coagulation dysfunction is a contraindication to performing lumbar puncture, but in some cases the risk of postponing LP outweighs the contraindication.
- Thrombocytopenia with platelet count above 40,000 probably does not pose a significant risk of bleeding complications from LP.
- Thrombocytopenia can be corrected with transfusion immediately before LP.
- Pharmacological anticoagulation usually can and should be corrected prior to LP.

Further Reading

Evans RW. Complications of lumbar puncture. *Neurol Clin*. 1998;16:83-105.

Hew-Wing P, Rolbin SH, Hew E, Amato D. Epidural anaesthesia and thrombocytopenia. *Anaesthesia*. 1989;44:775-777.

Sinclair AJ, Carroll C, Davies B. Cauda equina syndrome following a lumbar puncture. *J Clin Neurosci*. 2009;16:714-716.

van Veen JJ, Nokes TJ, Makris M. The risk of spinal haematoma following neuraxial anaesthesia or lumbar puncture in thrombocytopenic individuals. *Br J Haematol*. 2010;148:15.

6 Diffuse Weakness

In the ED a 28-year-old man complains of leg weakness
for the past day and a half. He thinks it might be due to
a strenuous rugby match 2 days before but feels that
things seem to be worsening. He denies headache, visual
problems, difficulty swallowing or breathing, but complains
about some pain in the posterior thighs and back. He has
had no bladder or bowel incontinence. He lives in a heavily
wooded area and wonders if his symtoms were caused by
a tick, despite noting no bites or rashes lately. He had a
"cold" 2 weeks ago. He has been diagnosed with bipolar
disorder and has been taking a combination of sodium
divalproex and sertraline over the past 6 months on the
advice of his psychiatrist. He also admits to frequent
marijuana use (to treat anxiety) and some alcohol use.
A first-year neurology resident has examined this patient
and found an entirely normal neurological exam including
mental status, cranial nerves, motor tone and strength,
sensation, and reflexes. You arrive in the ED and repeat
the exam and find all to be in order except for difficulty in
sitting up and even more difficulty climbing down to the
floor with some impairment in gait. Power in the upper
extremities is good, but the patient states that during this
assessment his arms "feel" weak. Reflexes are 2+ and
symmetrical. The patient's psychiatrist has been contacted
and suggests that conversion disorder is not likely.

What do you do now?

Although this case sounds like a standard presentation for Guillain-Barré syndrome (GBS), there are a few odd details. Given that the pathophysiology of GBS is thought to be an autoimmune attack on peripheral nerve myelin resulting from activation by an infectious agent (e.g., Campylobacter, Mycoplasma) with similar antigenic epitopes, a recent infection may be an important clue. Yet many patients with GBS cannot recall recent infections and the incidence of recent "colds" in the general population is probably high. Against the diagnosis might be the normal reflexes, sparing of the upper extremities, proximal location, and prominence of pain symptoms. On the other hand, GBS often begins with strictly leg weakness and even though distal sensory complaints are the rule, many patients do complain of back pain. And, reflexes may be normal for the first several days in GBS.

Other possibilities for subacute progressive weakness include myasthenia gravis, myasthenic syndrome (e.g., aminoglycoside-induced), tick paralysis, Lyme neuropathy, HIV polyradiculoneuropathy, hypercalcemia, hypokalemia, hypothyroidism, heavy metal intoxication (arsenic, lead, thallium), drugs (isoniazid [INH], vinca compounds, dapsone, nitrofurantoin), botulism, sarcoidosis, polymyositis, polio (highly unlikely in North America and Europe), and upper spinal cord lesions.

Myasthenia rarely begins in the proximal lower extremities and there is no history of instigators of a myasthenic syndrome in this patient. Botulism symptoms should include blurred vision. Polymyositis should be apparent on lab testing (with abnormatlities in creatine kinase [CK], erythrocyte sedimentation rate [ESR], CBC, and rheumatoid factor [RF]). Electrolyte abnormalities can easily be ruled out as can thyroid abnormalities and HIV infection. The patient was not taking medications known to cause generalized weakness. Lead neuropathy usually begins in the arms, and intoxication with arsenic and thallium usually causes gastrointestinal (GI) symptoms as well. Sarcoidosis can be ruled out to a reasonable extent with serum angiotensin converting enzyme titer and chest x-ray. CSF pleocytosis is also generally present in neurological sarcoid. Lyme disease can indeed cause a polyradiculitis, and the pathognomonic erythematous rash may have been missed, but cranial nerve palsies are much more common. Also, as with sarcoidosis, CSF pleocytosis is seen. Tick paralysis is, however, a real possibility as the patient has been exposed to the common causes—wood ticks and dog ticks. The presentation is similar to GBS, but CSF protein concentration should be normal. Tic paralysis is caused by a toxin that seems to interfere with acetylcholine release at the neuromuscular junction and abates soon after the tick is removed. Therefore a search for ticks is recommended, including the hair.

A common question is how far to proceed in searching for a spinal cord lesion in a patient such as this one. After all, he did play a highly physical sport the day symptoms began. The lack of reflex change or any bowel/bladder dysfunction argues against this etiology, but it is difficult to be sure in these cases, so cervical and thoracic spinal cord MRI (or even complete spinal MRI) might be reasonable here. A key test in this case is lumbar puncture to see whether CSF protein is high. Unfortunately, in the first week of GBS, around one-third of patients have normal CSF. Neurophysiological testing is often more fruitful early in the course of GBS with slowed motor conduction along with absent F and H waves.

So, despite a high clinical suspicion for the diagnosis of GBS, a number of mimics exist and workup needs to be thorough. Inpatient investigation is generally most convenient and efficient, and also provides the best setting to monitor the patient's neurological status, which is likely to worsen. Respiratory power should be monitored frequently with forced vital capacity (FVC) and negative inspiratory force (NIF), with a low threshold to consider elective intubation. If testing confirms GBS, intravenous immunoglobulin (IVIg) administration is generally begun unless symptoms are extremely mild. Plasma exchange is an alternative, but since it is more difficult and less available, IVIg has largely replaced it for the treatment of GBS in many institutions. Prognosis is generally very good for recovery, although the majority of patients will have some residual motor deficits.

KEY POINTS TO REMEMBER

- Acute Guillain-Barré syndrome may present in atypical fashion, without clear history of antecedent infection.
- The differential diagnosis in acute diffuse weakness is large with a number of entities producing similar symptomatology.
- A good initial workup of patients with acute weakness should include thorough metabolic screening as well as LP.
- Spinal imaging should be done early if there is any suspicion of myelopathy.

Further Reading

Fahoum F, Drory V, Issakov J, Neufeld MY. Neurosarcoidosis presenting as Guillain-Barre-like syndrome: a case report and review of the literature. *J Clin Neuromusc Dis.* 2009;11:35-43.

Krishnan AV, Lin CS, Reddel SW, Mcgrath R, Kiernan MC. Conduction block and impaired axonal function in tick paralysis. *Muscle Nerve.* 2009;40:358-362.

Vucica S, Kiernana MC, Cornblath DR. Guillain-Barré syndrome: an update. *J Clin Neurosci.* 2009;6:733-741.

7 Subacute Paraparesis in an Elderly Patient

An 81-year-old nursing home resident is brought to the ED by ambulance after a family member complained that he has become weak and unable to walk since the last visit 2 weeks ago. The patient agrees, but thinks it is just "stiffness" due to poor sleep. His caregiver attests to urinary incontinence and several occasions recently of fecal incontinence as well. He denies back or leg pain. He cannot remember any recent trauma. General exam reveals normal vital signs, normal lung and cardiac auscultation, and normal extremities. There is reduced range of motion in his neck but no spinal tenderness. Your exam reveals some cognitive deficits in memory, but reasonably good orientation, slow language, poor calculation, and some faulty judgment. The patient's daughter feels that his mental state seems to be at his recent baseline. There is good strength in the upper extremities but reduced power in the lower extremities in the 4-/5 range, particularly proximally in ileopsoas and hamstring muscles, with difficulty arising from the sitting position. Ambulation is impossible. Muscle stretch reflexes are reduced in the upper extremities and increased in the lower extremities. Abdominal reflexes are absent. Babinski reflexes are noted bilaterally along with 2-3 beats of clonus bilaterally. Sensation is reduced to light touch, pain, temperature, and vibration in both lower extremities below the mid-calf. Plain spinal films today reveal severe disc-space narrowing, arthropathy, and osteoporosis. CT scan of the head today reveals cortical atrophy and ventriculomegaly. A spine MRI from the preceding year reveals significant cervical and lumbar spinal stenosis with compression fractures at several levels. Recent brain MRI is remarkable for significant diffuse cortical atrophy; large lateral, third, and fourth ventricles; and several areas of subcortical white matter signal change.

What do you do now?

A number of medical issues are occurring simultaneously in this patient, as is often the case in his age group. First, and perhaps most important, he has a dementing illness or is acutely encephalopathic due to another cause. This will be important to understand as soon as possible, because diagnostic and treatment decisions differ dramatically for the two conditions. Dementia seems more likely given the chronicity of his mental status deficits, with Alzheimer's disease a probable cause. But the problems of most concern to caregivers are the loss of lower extremity power and incontinence. These, coupled with reflex abnormalities consistent with bilateral corticospinal tract dysfunction, suggest a lesion affecting the spinal cord. Loss of abdominal reflexes might support this as well, although loss of abdominal reflexes is not particularly diagnostic in this age group. The dissociation between strength in the upper and lower extremities speaks against a generalized process affecting motor tracts or nerves, and suggests a thoracic spinal cord locus.

A number of confounding issues, however, make it hard to interpret clues. Could the ventriculomegaly be more than just expansion of ventricular diameter due to cortical loss? Normal pressure hydrocephalus (NPH) can produce the cardinal symptoms this patient is currently manifesting: gait difficulty, incontinence, and cognitive decline. Could the hyper-reflexia be due to cervical spine disease with the level of myelopathy actually in the cervical cord? And the predominance of lower extremity symptoms be due to the more superficial layering of corticospinal tract fibers destined for lumbar and sacral segments? Sensation examination does not help us much, because there is no clear sensory level. In fact, the sensory loss in the distal lower extremities suggests polyneuropathy rather than central nervous system (CNS) dysfunction.

So what can the neurologist offer here? Even though last year's spinal MRI did not reveal a thoracic cord lesion, this patient could have developed a new lesion. A not uncommon scenario is a fall, with trauma to the back, leading to epidural hematoma. Once this is ruled out, the workup can proceed in a more measured fashion. Diagnostically, it also makes sense to use somatosensory evoked potentials (SSEP) to attempt to localize where the interruption in neural control might be. If lower extremity SSEP waveforms are markedly delayed, with relative sparing of upper extremity function, cervical myelopathy is less likely. If both are delayed, cervical spinal stenosis becomes a much more likely etiology, or is at least part of the problem.

There is considerable debate over when and how to operate on symptomatic cervical stenosis in the elderly. The anterior approach—discectomy with or without fusion—is more involved technically. The posterior approach—laminectomy—is associated with ultimately more deformity and perhaps more disability later. Osteopenia is a significant obstacle to both. As to the likelihood of return of function after surgery—hard to predict. But the level of disability these patients often experience makes taking a risk palatable given that nonsurgical methods are disappointing.

Another area where the neurologist can help is to lay the NPH diagnosis to rest, unless there is clear hydrocephalus out of proportion to the cortical atrophy, which, one suspects, is not the case here. Even in very suggestive cases, ventricular shunting often results in only modest improvement at best. A common misconception is that response to lumbar puncture with removal of large amounts of CSF can predict the outcome of shunting procedures. The major problem is that this "diagnostic" tap is fraught with a high frequency of false-negative and false-positive results. So LP is probably not indicated in this patient. An EEG is a reasonable test to order because recurrent epileptic seizures could certainly lead to incontinence and the appearance of cognitive decline. If not already checked recently, full metabolic and hematological screening including thyroid-function testing should also be done.

This patient's cognitive dysfunction is most likely the result of Alzheimer's disease in combination with subcortical ischemic disease. The family can be presented with the option of starting the patient on memantine or a cholinesterase inhibitor. Thiamine should be given, on the off-chance that there is an element of Wernicke's encephalopathy,which can certainly present with cognitive decline and gait dysfunction.

A hidden factor in this patient's presentation is the increasing care he is requiring. Incontinence alone amplifies the level of care he will need, and there are some living situations for which he is now ineligible, unless this problem improves. Likewise, his mental state implies that he will most likely be unable to do much self-care in the future, which, again, will require increased attention by caregivers. This sad progression is probably contributory to the visit to the ED today and will make decision-making even harder since admission to the hospital, even if there is some improvement in his status at discharge, may impact his return to his previous residence. The social work team should be notified as soon as possible so that all resources can be directed effectively.

KEY POINTS TO REMEMBER

- Gait dysfunction in the elderly is generally multifactorial.
- Acute spinal lesions must be identified and distinguished from chronic spondylitic and other conditions.
- The imaging assessment of normal pressure hydrocephalus hinges on the degree to which hydrocephalus is out of proportion to any expected "ex vacuo" ventriculomegaly due to brain atrophy.
- Quality-of-life issues become preeminent in the elderly age group and require sensitivity and a collaborative approach with family, caregivers, and social workers.

Further Reading

Marmarou A, Young HF, Aygok GA, et al. Diagnosis and management of idiopathic normal-pressure hydrocephalus: a prospective study in 151 patients. *J Neurosurg.* 2005;102(6):987-997.

Mummaneni PV, Kaiser MG, Matz PG, et al. Cervical surgical techniques for the treatment of cervical spondylotic myelopathy. *J Neurosurg Spine.* 2009;11:130-141.

Singh A, Crockard HA, Platts A, Stevens J. Clinical and radiological correlates of severity and surgery-related outcome in cervical spondylosis. *J. Neurosurg.* 2001;94:189-198.

8   Isolated Vertigo

A 69-year-old woman is seen in the ED for dizziness that
was first noted this morning when she woke up. She has
no other symptoms but is unable to walk. She describes
a sensation of movement and not knowing "which way
is up." She denies vision changes, trouble speaking,
sensory changes, and weakness. She does report mild
nausea when attempting to arise or walk. Her medical
history is remarkable for hypertension and borderline
diabetes. She had bilateral cataract surgery several
years ago. She denies a history of vertigo. General exam
reveals normal vital signs, a supple neck, clear lungs, and
normal cardiac exam. Neurological exam is remarkable
for midposition poorly reactive pupils, horizontal
nystagmus (worse on gaze to the left), and some gait
unsteadiness. Her speech is a bit dysarthric, but she
tells you this is due to her missing dentures. Strength
is normal. Reflexes are diffusely diminished. Sensation
is a bit reduced in her feet. Gait is unsteady, but base is
not widened. CT scan of the head reveals some cortical
atrophy and subtle white matter changes bilaterally.

What do you do now?

Sorting out the patient with "dizziness" can be tricky. The first step in evaluating these patients is to distinguish among the major symptoms that can lead a patient to complain of dizziness: (1) vertigo, (2) lightheadedness, and (3) disequilibrium. This is generally not difficult with an awake and articulate patient. However, when the patient has any degree of mental fogginess or anxiety (not uncommon), the distinctions become much more difficult. And, of course, there are a number of patients who use the word "dizzy" to refer to other perceptions such as confusion, visual change, clumsiness, or even anxiety.

Patients using the words "unbalanced," "wobbly," and "unsteady" are generally describing disequilibrium, which usually implicates cerebellar, cortico-cerebellar connections, or dorsal-column sensory dysfunction. CT scan of the head is a good initial step here, to rule out brainstem or cerebellar hemorrhage. An acute brainstem or cerebellar stroke will not be seen, however, so MRI is necessary to discover this. Generally, cerebrovascular causes of vertigo or imbalance will be accompanied by other signs of ischemia. A common cerebrovascular cause of vertigo is the Wallenberg syndrome, due to lateral medullary ischemia, which can consist of dysphagia, slurred speech, ataxia, ipsilateral facial sensation loss, contralateral body sensation loss, vertigo, nystagmus, Horner syndrome, and diplopia. In some cases, however, the ataxia and vertigo do predominate.

Patients who actually endorse a sensation of movement are probably feeling vertiginous, which implicates a lesion or lesions in labyrinths, vestibular nerves, or vestibular brainstem centers. Nausea is usually an accompaniment. Vestibular neuronitis or "labyrinthitis," thought to be a self-limited viral or otherwise inflammatory reaction in the labyrinthine system, is a common cause of vertigo at all ages. Again, posterior fossa hemorrhage or stroke should be considered. In cases of so-called "peripheral" vertigo (stemming from labyrinthine or vestibular nerve pathology) imaging will be negative, but the Dix-Hallpike maneuver should be positive with induction of severe vertigo (and probably nausea) when the extended head is turned to the side of the dysfunctional inner ear in the supine position. In addition, nystagmus (generally horizontal or diagonal rather than vertical) is brought on by this maneuver, but this can vary. Vestibular nerve involvement may be due to a mass in the cerebellopontine angle or an infectious/inflammatory process in the subarachnoid space affecting the acoustic nerve. Hence MRI and lumbar puncture are indicated if suspicion is high, particularly if other focal findings, such as cranial neuropathies, are seen on exam. Lyme titer, angiotensin converting enzyme level, and tests for syphilis are all worth considering in these cases. Electronystagmography can eventually confirm a labyrinthine cause of vertigo, but here cerebrovascular etiology is not entirely ruled out because small-vessel embolization (to the internal auditory artery or vestibular artery) or other occlusive pathophysiology can lead to essentially isolated vertigo. Other causes of vertigo include medications, Meniere's disease, perilymph fistula, and migraine (see Table 8.1).

TABLE 8.1 **Causes of Isolated Vertigo**

Benign positional vertigo

Medication effect—aspirin, nonsteroidal anti-inflammatory drugs, phenytoin, aminoglycosides

Vestibular neuronitis/Labyrinthitis

Meniere's disease

Post-traumatic vertigo

Phobic vertigo—situational

Perilymph fistula

Labyrinthine or brainstem ischemia

Meningitis—carcinomatous, tuberculous, fungal, bacterial

Ramsay Hunt syndrome (Zoster infec of Geniculate ganglion)

Brainstem or cerebellopontine region tumor

Complex partial seizures

Migraine

Multiple sclerosis—brainstem plaque

Brainstem neoplasm

Brainstem arteriovenous malformation (AVM)

Cogan's syndrome—autoimmune disease of inner ear

Arnold Chiari syndrome

Neurosyphilis—labyrinth infection, meningitis, arteritis

Intralabyrinthine hemorrhage (leukemia, trauma)

Sarcoidosis

Hyperventilation

Hypothyroidism

Hypoglycemia

Carcinoid syndrome

Cardiac arrhythmia

Pheochromocytoma

Vestibular neuronitis, unlike benign positional vertigo, is usually not *just* positional. Meniere's disease is eventually accompanied by hearing loss and/or tinnitus, but this may not yet be present. Perilymph fistula also generally involves a hearing loss, and there is almost always a history of an antecedent incident, such as weight lifting, barotrauma, scuba diving, or forceful nose-blowing. Meningeal infection or inflammation is usually suggested by meningismus, headache, or other cranial neuropathies. In migrainous vertigo there is usually a history of migraine, or at least a strong family history; coupling of symptoms with headache at least some of the time; and response to migraine abortive medications (e.g., triptans). Psychogenic vertigo can occur as well; clues include an absence of nystagmus and other neurological signs, and a history of phobias or panic attacks.

Lightheadedness is usually the term patients choose to describe presyncope, which is generally related to some reduction in cerebral perfusion. This can be due to any number of conditions, ranging from dehydration to a serious cardiovascular condition (see Chapter 9—Syncope). Workup should begin with a thorough cardiovascular exam and an electrocardiogram. More lengthy cardiac monitoring, echocardiography, and imaging of the cervical arteries with CT or MRI angiography may be necessary as well. Tilt table testing may be indicated if autonomic instability is suspected.

This patient seems to have more than just vertigo—although virtually all of her other symptoms may have a benign explanation—the dysarthria may indeed be due to her dental issues, the pupillary unreactivity is probably related to cataract surgery, and the gait difficulty may be entirely due to vertigo and/or peripheral neuropathy. So a labyrinthine cause of vertigo, like vestibular neuronitis, is likely. But she has risk factors for stroke and is in an age group where this is more probable—so she should probably be admitted at least for observation while workup is pending. One should be prepared for a negative workup, however, because cerebrovascular causes of isolated vertigo are actually infrequent.

Despite the cause, vertigo can be treated reasonably well with anticholinergics or antihistamines. Many patients find oral or parenteral hydroxyzine to be helpful, and for severe vertigo, transdermal scopolamine is very effective. If migrainous vertigo is suspected, a trial of a triptan (if cerebro- and cardiovascular disease has been ruled out) may be very useful.

- "Dizziness" can indicate any of several different perceptual states including vertigo, imbalance, and lightheadedness.
- In patients who have risk factors for cardiovascular and cerebrovascular disease, an initial CT scan, and later MRI, cerebral vascular imaging, and echocardiography are probably indicated.
- Vertigo, when accompanied by cranial neuropathies, should prompt lumbar puncture if there are no contraindications.
- Lightheadedness with or without syncope should lead to cardiac evaluation.

Further Reading

Grad A, Baloh RW. Vertigo of vascular origin: clinical and electronystagmographic features in 84 Cases. *Arch Neurol.* 1989;46:281-284.

Kerber KA, Brown DL, Lisabeth LD, et al. Stroke among patients with dizziness, vertigo, and imbalance in the emergency department: a population-based study. *Stroke.* 2006;37:2484-2487.

Neuhauser H, Lempert T. Vertigo and dizziness related to migraine: a diagnostic challenge. *Cephalalgia.* 2004;24:83-91.

9 Syncope

A 68-year-old woman had a loss of consciousness at home yesterday afternoon. She admitted this to her daughter this morning when asked about the cut on her head. She further admitted to several ("maybe half a dozen") previous episodes of loss of consciousness, some of which led to falls, over the past three to four years. She feels fine now, although she is anxious. She denies incontinence of urine or feces. She did experience a mild headache when recovering from her syncopal attack yesterday, but "it's gone now." Her medical history includes mild chronic obstructive pulmonary disease (COPD) and controlled hypertension. Her BP now is 148/78, does not drop significantly on sitting or standing (142/76 sitting, 146/70 standing), and her pulse is 88 and regular. Respirations are 14 per minute and she is afebrile. Neurological exam is intact including mental status, cranial nerves, strength, reflexes, coordination, and gait. She asks you why this happened and worries about the possibility of it happening again, "maybe even when I am driving!"

What do you do now?

The conscious patient reporting syncope is one of the most frequent triggers for both neurological and cardiological consultation in the ED. The first step is to determine if, in fact, this was syncope (brief loss of consciousness). Some patients will ultimately be found to have had transient loss of vision, lightheadedness (presyncope), or transient confusion. If it seems likely there was a transient loss of consciousness, and this can be corroborated by witnesses or perhaps by evidence of trauma sustained during a fall, which often accompanies syncope, the next step is to attempt to discover clues to the loss of consciousness. Table 9.1 lists causes of loss of consciousness, which include those due to reduced cardiac output (and consequent blood flow to the brain), hypoglycemia, hypoxia, cerebrovascular events, and seizure.

In the case above, stroke is unlikely, as neurological exam is normal, and hemorrhage has been ruled out by negative CT of the head. Posterior cerebral circulation occlusive disease is possible, but is unlikely in the absence

TABLE 9.1 **Causes of Brief Loss of Consciousness**

Cardiac arrhythmia
Myocardial infarction
Pericarditis or cardiac tamponade
Cardiomyopathy
Aortic stenosis
Mitral valve stenosis or prolapse or atrial myxoma
Dissecting aortic aneurysm
Orthostatic hypotension
Pneumothorax
Pulmonary stenosis
Pulmonary hypertension
Pulmonary embolus
Basilar artery occlusion
Stroke
Subclavian steal syndrome
Intracerebral or subarachnoid hemorrhage
Carotid sinus syncope
Hypoglycemia
Anemia
Hypoxemia
Hypercarbia
Vasovagal syncope
Psychogenic syncope

of typical accompanying symptoms, such as vertigo, imbalance, dysarthria, facial numbness, or visual loss. MRI of the brain, as well as vascular imaging (either MR or CT angiography), can help to exclude this.

Intermittent arrhythmias that reduce cardiac output can be occult, but cardiac-rhythm monitoring, via inpatient telemetry, or portable monitoring system, generally clarifies the presence of this as a cause. BP should be checked in both arms to investigate the possibility of subclavian stenosis/coarctation leading perhaps to subclavian steal. A strong clue to this pathophysiology is instigation of syncope by exercise of the ipsilateral arm (promoting "stealing" of blood from the brain via the vertebral artery to supply the arm). Chest x-ray and echocardiography should be done to rule out pericarditis, tamponade, mitral valve, aortic valve or atrial pathology, and cardiomyopathy. Hypotension, venous engorgement, weak pulse, and findings on cardiac auscultation might also be present with cardiac disease.

Orthostatic hypotension (OH) should be relatively straightforward to rule out. A drop in diastolic pressure of more than 10 mm Hg or systolic of 20 mm, when the patient sits or stands up, is diagnostic. If orthostatic tachycardia occurs, one suspects hypovolemia; if not, there may be an element of dysautonomia. The potential causes of OH include drug effects (e.g.anticholinergics, dopaminergics, or diuretics), autonomic neuropathies (e.g., diabetes or amyloid neuropathy), Parkinson's disease and "Parkinson-plus" syndromes (multisystem atrophy), hypovolemia, and anemia. If OH is identified, these should all be investigated.

Vasovagal syncope, also referred to as neurocardiogenic syncope, is caused by a relative surge in parasympathetic activity, precipitated by emotional stress, fear, excessive coughing, pain, or in some cases urination (micturition syncope). Bradycardia and hypotension lead to brain hypoperfusion. Premonitory symptoms can include diaphoresis, pallor, and nausea. This may be the most common cause of syncope and is essentially a diagnosis of exclusion until the patient notices a pattern of recurrence in identical situations. When vasovagal syncope results from autonomic hypersensitivity to position changes it begins to resemble orthostatic hypotension. Using a tilt table to incline the patient during monitoring for BP and pulse rate can be diagnostic. Treatment includes avoidance of triggers, volume expansion tactics, and medications.

Chest or abdominal pain and/or dyspnea should be present to at least some degree in myocardial infarction, pneumothorax, dissecting aortic aneurysm, and pulmonary embolism. Measuring levels of cardiac enzymes should be considered. Anemia, hypoxemia, hypercarbia, and other metabolic disturbances can be easily ruled out with routine labs and pulse oximetry. Carotid sinus syncope occurs when the carotid sinus is compressed by a tight collar, a seat belt or backpack strap, or other source of external pressure. This results in vagal stimulation leading to bradycardia and vasodilation with resulting systemic hypotension.

Seizures, when generalized, cause loss of consciousness. A key to the diagnosis here is postictal alteration of mentation, consciousness, or focal neurological function. Patients tend to recover pretty quickly after cardiovascular syncope. Other important clues are witness reports of motor movements, evidence of tongue biting, and incontinence. Interestingly, causes of syncope that lead to some degree of cerebral hypoxia can briefly cause tonic clonic movements, mimicking epileptic seizures.

Drug intoxication is always a possibility, although a classic syncopal event is unlikely. Still, drug screening must be considered. Psychogenic syncope is seen in patients with depression, anxiety, and panic. Vasovagal mechanisms, hyperventilation, or somatization may be the proximate cause in these patients.

So, there are a number of possibilities here, including several relatively unlikely neurological ones. The neurologist who can reason through these cases and offer advice other than "order an EEG" will be much respected and appreciated.

KEY POINTS TO REMEMBER

- Syncope can result from many causes including cardiovascular, pulmonary, metabolic, neurological, and psychogenic.
- Careful general, cardiac, pulmonary, and neurological history and exams are essential, including careful assessment of pulse and blood pressure bilaterally and in different positions.
- Laboratory investigation of syncope should include metabolic and hematological panels, and cardiac enzymes. ECG, chest x-ray, EEG, echocardiography, and cardiac monitoring should be part of the investigation as well.
- Cerebrovascular imaging should likewise be considered in cases of syncope accompanied by any focal neurological deficits or when there is a suspicion of seizure.

Further Reading

Chen-Scarabelli C, Scarabelli TM. Neurocardiogenic syncope. *BMJ.* 2004;329: 336-341.

Moya A, Sutton R, Ammirati F, et al. Guidelines for the diagnosis and management of syncope. *Eur Heart J.* 2009;30:2631-2671.

Serrano LA, Hess EP, Bellolio MF, et al. Accuracy and quality of clinical decision rules for syncope in the emergency department: a systematic review and meta-analysis. *Ann Emerg Med.* 2010;56:362-373.

10 Acute Monocular Visual Loss

A 46-year-old laboratory technician is seen for acute
visual loss in the right eye. She states that vision seemed
normal the day before. General exam is normal—vital
signs are normal; neck is supple; lungs, heart, and
abdomen are normal; there is no skin rash. Routine labs
are normal. Ocular exam is normal, without papilledema,
but pupillary reactivity to light is sluggish on the
right with a Marcus Gunn pupil. Neurological exam is
essentially normal with no cranial nerve abnormalities.

What do you do now?

Acute vision loss is a daunting presentation. Rapid identification of the cause and speedy corrective measures are imperative. Fortunately for neurologists, the answers are usually clarified by ophthalmologists, but a common reason for consultation arises when "ocular causes have been ruled out."

The differential diagnosis of acute monocular vision loss can be divided into the following categories, beginning with the most peripheral and moving more centrally:

1. Opacities in the cornea, lens, or vitreous humour
2. Retinal disease
3. Retinal or eye ischemia
4. Optic nerve disease, ischemic or demyelinating
5. Disease of the chiasm
6. Conversion, factitious or malingering

Ocular opacities such as corneal edema or vitreous hemorrhage generally do not cause a deafferented pupil even with dramatic visual blurring or loss. And they are generally painless. Funduscopic exam is generally diagnostic when done by a competent ophthalmologist. Iritis and uveitis can obscure vision due to localized edema, but eye pain and obvious ocular inflammation generally lead these patients to where they need to be—into the hands of an ophthalmologist. Acute retinal detachment usually is painless and begins with some degree of vitreous detachment with patients complaining of "floaters." Retinal detachment may eventually cause a Marcus Gunn pupil. Complaints usually begin with peripheral field loss. Regular funduscopic exam is often negative, although occasionally one can see the classic white "billowing" retinal separation. A dilated eye exam by an ophthalmologist is usually positive.

Ischemia of the retina can arise in the setting of several different disease states. Amaurosis fugax (transient loss of vision in one eye), often occurs usually in the form of a "shade coming down" and then receding. This generally arises as the result of atherosclerotic or thrombotic emboli to the central retinal artery, or one of its retinal branches, from a diseased carotid artery. Occasionally, one can see small atheromatous or calcific fragments in retinal arteries on funduscopic exam. If the embolus remains lodged long enough, retinal ischemic injury can occur and lead to permanent visual impairment.

Retinal artery occlusion may cause deafferentation. Funduscopic exam usually reveals an area of paleness on the retina with a red macula due to its thinner epithelium. There is little or no effective treatment for this condition, although hydration, assurance of optimal carotid system perfusion, and perhaps ocular massage may help. Searching for the specific etiology and treatment of it is, of course, imperative in hopes of preventing further CNS ischemia. More proximal embolic or atheromatous occlusion of the ophthalmic artery may also cause monocular vision loss, and can, like strokes elsewhere, occur on the basis of cardiac, paradoxical, or arterial embolization; arterial thrombosis; or atherosclerotic narrowing.

Central retinal vein occlusion is another fairly frequent cause of acute monocular vision loss and is generally diagnosed funduscopically by observing multiple retinal hemorrhages and papilledema. The associated vision loss is often not as severe as that resulting from arterial occlusion. Best treatment is not clear, but most cases seem to be self-limited. Temporal arteritis (TA, or Giant-cell arteritis, GCA) affects the temporal artery and extradural portions of the carotid and vertebral arteries. This includes the ophthalmic artery so visual loss can occur as a result of resulting ischemia to the retina and/or optic nerve. TA usually presents with severe headache and often with polymyalgia rheumatica, and occasionally one can detect a tender temporal artery. By the time vision has been impaired it is probably too late to save what has been lost, but rapid treatment with intravenous steroids can prevent further loss. Retinal vasculitis can also produce monocular visual impairment, and is diagnosed with dilated funduscopic exam and flourescein angiography. The condition is usually painless. Etiology is often not discovered, but management consists of searching for systemic causes of vasculitis and treatment with immunosuppressants.

Anterior ischemic optic neuropathy generally occurs in patients with diabetes, hypertension, or lupus. Papilledema is often seen. Treatment is aimed at the underlying disease(s) and patients often improve. Optic neuritis (ON) due to acute demyelination is often painful and usually causes a deafferentated pupil early, along with the vision loss. Papilledema is seen when the inflammation is close to the retina, but when it is retrobulbar, diagnosis rests on clinical suspicion along with brain MRI findings of demyelination in the parenchyma. Also, enhanced MRI can reveal optic nerve inflammation. Standard treatment of ON is IV methylprednisolone.

Optic neuritis can be seen as an isolated syndrome (although there is a significant chance of developing MS), as an exacerbation of MS, or as the presentation of neuromyelitis optica (NMO) or Devic's disease. Leber optic neuropathy is inherited mitochondrially and can lead to unilateral optic neuropathy either subacutely or acutely. Eventual involvement of the other eye is the rule. There is no known treatment.

Mass lesions or infections affecting the optic nerve in the orbit or in the region of optic foramen generally progress more slowly with gradual visual impairment over weeks or longer. Involvement of the optic chiasm by neoplastic and infectious disease does not lead to monocular vision loss but rather to bitemporal or homonymous field deficits.

Conversion disorder may cause monocular blindness, but it is more often binocular and can be detected fairly easily by normal optokinetic strip testing, normal visual evoked potentials, or by its nonanatomic features. Partial visual field loss due to malingering or factitious disorder is more difficult to detect, although clinical suspicion should be high when secondary gain is obvious.

Diagnostic workup, once thorough ophthalmological examination has been done and found to be normal, should include the following: complete blood count, erythrocyte sedimentation rate (ESR), C-reactive protein, antinuclear antibody, hemoglobin A1c, brain MRI, MR angiogram and/ or carotid ultrasound, and echocardiogram. If suspicion for demyelinating disease is high, NMO antibody should be checked. If the diagnosis is not clear, Lyme titer, HIV screen, LP with CSF exam to include protein, glucose, fungal and tubercle bacilli stains and cultures, and oligoclonal bands should be done.

KEY POINTS TO REMEMBER

- Ophthalmological evaluation is critical in acute monocular visual loss, and should include a dilated funduscopic exam (*prior to which careful pupillary testing should be done*).
- When ophthalmological causes of monocular blindness have been excluded, retinal ischemia, ischemic optic neuritis, and demyelinating optic neuritis must be considered.
- Diagnostic testing in acute visual loss should include brain and vascular imaging, ESR, and possibly lumbar puncture.

Further Reading

Lennon VA, Wingerchuk DM, Kryzer TJ, et al. A serum autoantibody marker of neuromyelitis optica: distinction from multiple sclerosis. *Lancet.* 2004;364:2106-2112.

Schmidt D. Ocular massage in a case of central retinal artery occlusion—the successful treatment of a hitherto undescribed type of embolism. *Eur J Med Res.* 2000;5:157-164.

Vortmann M, Schneider JI. Acute monocular visual loss. *Emerg Med Clin North Am.* 2008;26:73-96.

Ward TN, Levin M. Headache in giant cell arteritis and other arteritides. *Neurol Sci.* 2005; 26(suppl 2):s134-s137.

11 Thunderclap Headache

A 37-year-old woman developed a severe headache while biking up a challenging hill. She had to get off her bike, and then she called 911, which led to her arrival in the ED by ambulance. She told the ED staff that she has never had headaches, and that this one "made me see stars." She continues, 2 hours after the onset of this headache, to be in pain and also has blurred vision. CT of the head, and LP, have both been done and are entirely negative. General and neurological exams are normal.

What do you do now?

This, of course, is the famous "thunderclap headache." Most patients will seek attention and some will turn out to have one of the scarier conditions known to cause sudden severe headaches, such as intracerebral hemorrhage or subarachnoid hemorrhage, which are identified with CT and LP (See Table 11.1—Causes of Thunderclap Headache). Seeing "stars" and complaining of persistent visual difficulties are clues that there may indeed be an underlying secondary cause of headache here. So—what is a wise course of action when this initial workup is negative? One problem is that several causes of thunderclap headache are identifiable only with more advanced imaging. Cerebral venous thrombosis is one example; standard MRI imaging may fail to identify even large thrombi in cerebral veins. MR or CT venography, however, is almost always diagnostic. The syndrome of reversible cerebral vasoconstriction syndrome (RCVS), also known as "Call-Fleming syndrome," often presents as sudden or severe headache and only later manifests neurological deficits. Unlike CNS vasculitis, CSF in RCVS is generally normal and MRI is often normal as well. The hallmark of RCVS is segmental arterial narrowing seen on angiography. Fortunately, CT angiography seems to be almost as useful as standard intra-arterial angiography. Interestingly, RCVS often becomes symptomatic (with severe headache) after vigorous exercise, and may well be the explanation for this patient's presentation. To complicate matters, RCVS may lead to focal subarachnoid bleeding, which can lead to a fruitless quest for a ruptured aneurysm. While in most cases RCVS is a self-limited disorder, calcium channel blockers are often used in some centers to prevent stroke.

TABLE 11.1   **Causes of Sudden (Thunderclap) Headache**

- Subarachnoid hemorrhage or "aneurysmal leak" (sentinel headache)
- Hypertensive, lobar, or pituitary intracranial hemorrhage
- Cerebral venous thrombosis
- Carotid or vertebral artery dissection
- Intracranial hypotension
- Cerebral vasculitis
- Reversible cerebral vasoconstriction syndrome (RCVS)
- Acute hypertension
- Primary thunderclap headache
- Sphenoid sinusitis

Carotid or vertebral arterial dissection can present with acute severe headache and without other neurological symptoms. Again, vascular imaging, including the proximal segments of these vessels, is required for exclusion of dissection. Sphenoid sinusitis may also present as sudden diffuse head pain, and although it may be missed on CT, MRI is generally quite adequate to diagnose it. Spontaneous intracranial hypotension, generally diagnosed by the patient's complaint of worsening of pain upon sitting or standing and improvement with reclining, may present with thunderclap headache. Exertional headaches are generally short-lived, but exercise-induced migraine may persist, similar to regular migraine, for hours or even days. Likewise, orgasmic headaches, thought to represent a benign primary headache type, can persist and mimic serious vascular causes. A key distinguishing feature, of course, is that these follow a pattern—stereotypic, recurring, sudden (or at least rapidly escalating) global headaches at or near the time of orgasm—and orgasmic headache has probably never been reported to occur while biking. Finally, a primary benign headache condition termed "benign thunderclap headache" presents in this way, and is obviously a diagnosis of exclusion.

But have we really excluded berry aneurysm as an underlying cause of this patient's severe acute headache? Head CT imaging resolution is generally considered adequate to detect subarachnoid blood. Some reports suggest, however, that between 1% and 5% of results are false negatives. Hence, the need for lumbar puncture, but it, too, has a finite false-positive rate, particularly if the hemorrhage was recent, deep,and/or limited. There have been several reports of patients with *unruptured* aneurysms, or aneurysms that have "leaked," and produced thunderclap headaches (so-called "sentinel headaches") without producing bloody CSF. MRI is generally very sensitive to even small amounts of subarachnoid blood, undetectable by CT or in the CSF sample, but high resolution cerebrovascular imaging is necessary to exclude the possibility of an unruptured aneurysm. The mechanism underlying acute headache with unruptured aneurysm is not clear, but some have postulated stretching of the nociceptive receptors in the aneurysmal wall as causal. The International Classification of Headache Disorders also included unruptured arteriovenous malformations as a cause of headache, but these are generally not thunderclap in presentation.

So, what is the most parsimonious workup for thunderclap headache once CT and LP have emerged negative? A brain MRI to rule out recent hemorrhage, MRA of the cerebral vessels to investigate for aneurysm (or AVM) and segmental arterial narrowing, MRA of the cervical vessels to look for dissection, and an MR venogram to rule out cerebral venous thrombosis would be a very thorough approach. MR angiography may not be as sensitive as CT angiography for detecting berry aneurysms, so this, or a conventional intra-arterial dye angiogram should be considered.

If all serious causes of thunderclap headache are ruled out, Primary Thunderclap Headache may be the diagnosis, although it must be viewed with suspicion. Indomethacin may relieve this type of headache, but opioids may be necessary.

KEY POINTS TO REMEMBER

- Sudden severe headache is a potential emergency and should be evaluated with CT and, if negative, LP to rule out hemorrhage.
- Several diagnostic possibilities for thunderclap headache may not be diagnosed with CT, LP, or even MRI.
- Primary thunderclap headache, thought to be a primary headache disorder, may be the underlying diagnosis but must be a diagnosis of exclusion.

Further Reading

Day JW, Raskin NH. Thunderclap headache: symptom of unruptured cerebral aneurysm. *Lancet*. 1986;2(8518):1247-1248.

Kowalski RG, Claassen J, Kreiter KT, et al. Initial misdiagnosis and outcome after subarachnoid hemorrhage. *JAMA*. 2004;291:866-869.

Singhal AB. Diagnostic challenges in RCVS, PACNS, and other cerebral arteriopathies. *Cephalalgia*. 2011;31:1067-1070.

Febrile Delirium with Rigidity

A 42-year-old man with schizophrenia was found today in his supervised-living dormitory room by a caretaker, confused, somnolent, and "feeling hot." Apparently he looked a little "down" yesterday and did not eat much, but was seen to be normal otherwise. He is not verbally responsive in the ED but is breathing regularly. His temperature is 40° C and his BP is 160/100. He is tachycardic at 120. There are no rashes, neck is supple, lungs are clear, no murmurs are auscultated, and the abdomen is flat and non-tender. Neurological exam, other than mental status, is nonfocal. White blood cell count (WBC) is elevated at 16,000. CK is markedly elevated at 10,500.

What do you do now?

Neuroleptic medications can induce several neurological syndromes: (1) acute dystonia, (2) akathisia, (3) oculogyric crisis, (4) parkinsonism, (5) tardive dyskinesia, and (6) neuroleptic malignant syndrome (NMS). This patient's presentation is typical for NMS—encephalopathy, hyperthermia, muscle rigidity, tachycardia, and elevated CK—but other possibilities must be considered. Encephalitis can look similar but for the muscle rigidity and CK elevation. Drugs such as cocaine and amphetamines (including 3,4-methylenedioxymethamphetamine, or MDMA) and other toxins can produce an encephalopathy and fever, as do some withdrawal syndromes including ethanol. But again, the very high CK would be odd, unless the patient had sustained trauma on such a level as to cause significant muscle breakdown. Status epilepticus can elevate CK but not to these levels. Other possibilities include malignant hyperthermia, serotonin syndrome, anticholinergic overdose, and rabies.

Malignant hyperthermia is a genetic disorder resulting from ryanodine receptor mutations, which presents with fever, rigidity, tremors, agitated delirium, and hallucinosis, and progresses to stupor and coma. It is generally provoked by inhalation anesthetics and/or depolarizing muscle relaxants. Treatment consists of cooling, dantrolene sodium (a direct-acting muscle relaxant) 1-to-2 mg/kg IV in repeated doses, and bicarbonate to normalize metabolic acidosis. Arrhythmias must be treated and electrolyte imbalances corrected. Malignant hyperthermia can be difficult to differentiate from NMS, so history is crucial.

Serotonin syndrome (SS), due usually to additive effects of multiple serotonergic medications (e.g., SSRI with a monoamine oxidase [MAO] inhibitor), manifests with many of the same features, but is usually accompanied by hyper-reflexia as opposed to NMS which usually causes hyporeflexia. Also, patients with SS usually do not have an elevated WBC count. Treatment consists of serotonin blockers such as methysergide or cyproheptadine.

The viral encephalitis of rabies resembles NMS a bit more than herpes simplex or other viral encephalitides. Patients can present with the "furious" form with fever, agitation, motor hyperactivity, hallucinosis, confusion, and ultimately seizures and coma. There can be calm (lucid) periods. Rigidity is unlikely, however, and creatine phosphokinase (CPK) does not rise nearly as high as in NMS. There is a less common form in which paralysis of limbs is an early manifestation. While it is uncommon to contract rabies from an infected human, precautions must be observed if it is suspected.

Overdose with anticholinergic medication, including cyclic antidepressants and antihistamines, can present with febrile encephalopathy. Presentation can include fever, tachycardia, hypotension, encephalopathy, and muscle rigidity. Skin is usually dry and the patient has mydriasis.

So, diagnosis in cases of delirium with hyperthermia, such as the one here, can be challenging, with overlapping symptoms and signs seen in several conditions (Tables 12.1 and 12.2). Diagnostic approaches should include CT of the head, LP with CSF analysis including viral PCR testing, EEG, CBC, full chemistry panel, toxicology screen, urine myoglobin, lactate levels, arterial blood gases, and blood cultures.

One of the pitfalls in diagnosing NMS is that in the early stages patients can be misinterpreted to be worsening in terms of their psychiatric condition and be treated with higher doses of neuroleptic medication, when in fact, stopping neuroleptic treatment is essential. The syndrome can be initiated by chronic neuroleptic use, or even shortly after beginning neuroleptic medication, but there has to have been some use within the last 3 days. NMS can also be induced by cessation of dopaminergic medication such as L-Dopa or bromocriptine. Cessation of baclofen can also induce NMS. The classic symptomatology includes confusion and later agitated delirium, tremor, and hallucinations. Exam reveals rigidity, tremor, spasms, confusion, and fever. Treatment consists of cooling, dantrolene sodium 1-to-2 mg/kg

TABLE 12.1 **Differential Diagnosis of Hyperthermia with Delirium**

Meningitis–generally bacterial

Viral encephalitis

Rabies

Malignant hyperthermia

Neuroleptic malignant syndrome

Serotonin syndrome

Anticholinegic medication overdose

Status epilepticus

Drug overdose–cocaine, amphetamines

Drug, ethanol withdrawal

TABLE 12.2 **Comparison of Presentation in Serotonin Syndrome, Neuroleptic Malignant Syndrome, Malignant Hyperthermia, and Anticholinergic Overdose**

Symptom/ sign	Serotonin syndrome	NMS	Malignant hyperthermia	Anticholinergic toxicity
Delirium	+	+	+	+
Fever	+	+	+	+
Autonomic dysfunction	+	+	+	+
Pupils	dilated			dilated
Nausea/ vomiting	+			
Rigidity	+	+	+	+
Reflexes	increased	decreased	decreased	
Clonus	+			
Tremor	+			
CK	high	high	high	
Treatment	benzodiazepine, cyproheptadine, antihistamine	bromocriptine, dantrolene, benzodiazepine	dantrolene	

IV, repeated every few hours, and bromocriptine 2.5-to-10 mg tid. Volume depletion must be corrected with IV fluids. Hypotension may also respond to fluid boluses. Cooling methods include cooling blankets, ice packs, cold IV fluids, and antipyretics. When rhabdomyolysis occurs, hydration and alkalinization of the urine with sodium bicarbonate is essential in hopes of

KEY POINTS TO REMEMBER

- Febrile encephalopathy is a dire emergency that requires a speedy workup and may require empiric antibiotic treatment while diagnostic tests are pending.
- Muscle rigidity and high CK in the setting of febrile encephalopathy are suggestive of NMS.
- Treatment of NMS includes hydration, cooling, muscle relaxation, and immediate cessation of all neuroleptic medications.

preventing renal failure. Benzodiazepines can also help reduce muscle rigidity. Prognosis in NMS was said to be poor in the past but more recently, with proper care, at least 90% of patients will survive.

Further Reading

Strawn JR, Keck PE Jr, Caroff SN. Neuroleptic malignant syndrome. *Am J Psychiatry.* 2007;164:870-876.

Gurrera RJ, Caroff SN, Cohen A, Carroll BT, DeRoos F, Francis A. An international consensus study of neuroleptic malignant syndrome diagnostic criteria using the Delphi method. *J Clin Psychiatry.* 2011;72:1222-1228.

Odagaki Y. Atypical neuroleptic malignant syndrome or serotonin toxicity associated with atypical antipsychotics?. *Curr Drug Saf.* 2009;4:84-93.

PART II

Therapeutic Dilemmas in Adult Patients

13 Acute Stroke after 3 Hours

A 59-year-old man with untreated hypertension began having difficulty moving his right arm approximately 3 hours ago and soon afterward found that his speech was impaired as well. Both symptoms have persisted. He denies any other new problems, but earlier he did experience transient headache, now resolved. The patient is entirely alert, has some difficulty speaking, but is not dysarthric, has decreased movement in his face below the eyes on the right, and clearly has trouble using his right arm. Mental status exam is essentially normal, but speech fluency is reduced, and there are several phonemic paraphasic errors. Paresis is noted in the right deltoid, triceps, biceps, wrist extensors, and finger extensors in the 4/5 range. Sensation seems intact. Coordination and gait seem intact. CT of the head is negative, ECG shows sinus rhythm without any signs of cardiac ischemia. His wife pleads with you to do something as he is a carpenter and they are very worried about a disabling stroke.

What do you do now?

It is quite possible that this couple has heard about new "life-saving" (or disability-preventing) treatments for acute stroke. Tissue plasminogen activator (tPA, alteplase) is not FDA-approved for use in stroke of longer than 3 hours duration. So, nothing to do, right? Actually, in many cases of acute stroke that presumably occurred more than the magical 3 hours ago, there are several interventional options. This, of course, is a case where all reasonable interventions should be considered—aphasia and right-arm weakness in a young active patient—so you will want to explore these with this patient in a timely way.

When researchers looked carefully at data from the third European Cooperative Acute Stroke Study (ECASS III) of tPA in stroke, it became apparent that for patients who are not anticoagulated, who do not have both a history of diabetes and previous stroke, who are under 80 years of age, and who are not beyond 4½ hours from the onset of symptoms, intravenous tPA may actually be of significant help. The other exclusionary criteria should be used, including large stroke (NIH stroke scale > 25). So, if patients are willing, tPA can be given IV in cases like this one. Data that might help make these decisions easier can be obtained from perfusion CT or MR studies, which can identify cerebral tissue at risk of ischemia and therefore theoretically salvageable. With large at-risk areas, later attempts at thrombolysis become more attractive.

Alternatively, the option of dissolving the thrombus more directly may appeal to you and your patient. Intra-arterial tPA carries additional risks, particularly intracerebral hemorrhage, but may be effective in dramatically restoring function in some patients. Hemorrhages can occur because of vessel perforation by the catheter, but other possible causes are reperfusion-induced high flow and blood pressure fluctuations during the procedure. The prerequisites include CT exclusion of hemorrhage and tumors, vascular imaging to identify thrombus location, moderate size of stroke with stable findings, controlled blood pressure, and, most important, an experienced neuroradiological interventionalist in your institution who is ready to catheterize and infuse. The time window here is considered to be longer: 6 hours with stroke in the anterior circulation and up to 24 hours for posterior-circulation stroke. So this option may be very attractive when the timing is not right for IV thrombolysis. There have been several trials of IV, followed by intra-arterial tPA administration. The ultimate results do not support better long-term outcomes so this is not done in most institutions.

Finally, if the option is available in your institution, clot "extraction" can be attempted. Unfortunately this is still experimental and carries some risk even in the best of hands. The key prerequisite is vascular imaging that identifies occlusion but no arterial dissection. Here, there are several technical options. The Merci device comes in different diameters based on the diameter of the vessel involved, and includes a balloon proximally, aimed at dilating the artery, and a corkscrew portion distally, designed to capture the clot and ultimately extract it while suction is applied. The Penumbra devices are also sized, and consist of a probe that pierces the thrombus, and a sheath ("separator") that is designed to disengage the clot from the luminal wall, encase it, and then extract it. The Penumbra device also uses suction as the clot is extracted. The Solitaire "flow restoration" device uses a stent to encircle the thrombus, and extract it via suctioning. Revascularization is achieved at a high rate with all of these approaches, although, as might be imagined, risks are higher than with less invasive options. Often, intra-arterial chemical thrombolysis (with tPA) is combined with mechanical thrombus extraction.

So, this case of apparent acute left-hemispheric anterior-circulation stroke presents some opportunities, if evaluation and decisions can be made quickly. Vascular imaging (e.g., with CT angiography) might well identify an intra-arterial thrombus, which can be treated with IV or intra-arterial tPA. If this is ineffective, or if the patient is interested in a more aggressive approach, mechanical thrombus extraction can be attempted, if this technology and the appropriate radiological interventionalist are available. If there is time, MR perfusion sequences can provide information about at-risk cerebral tissue, which then can inform these decisions.

KEY POINTS TO REMEMBER

- The third European Cooperative Acute Stroke Study (ECASS III) suggests a longer time window for good results with IV tPA in a large subgroup of patients.
- Intra-arterial tPA can be a good choice when the site of thrombosis is identified, with an even longer time window.
- Mechanical clot extraction technology has advanced to the point where it, too, deserves serious consideration for a number of acute-stroke patients.

Further Reading

Adams HP, del Zoppo G, Alberts MJ. Guidelines for the Early Management of Adults with Ischemic Stroke. A Guideline from the American Heart Association/American Stroke Association Stroke Council, Clinical Cardiology Council, Cardiovascular Radiology and Intervention Council, and the Atherosclerotic Peripheral Vascular Disease and Quality of Care Outcomes in Research Interdisciplinary Working Groups. *Stroke.* 2007;38:1655-1711.

Hacke W, Kaste M, Bluhmki E, et al. Thrombolysis with alteplase 3 to 4.5 hours after acute ischemic stroke. *N Engl J Med.* 2008;359:1317-1329.

Samaniego EA, Linfante I, Dabus G. Intra-arterial thrombolysis: tissue plasminogen activator and other thrombolytic agents. *Tech Vasc Interv Radiol.* 2012;15:41-46.

Tenser MS, Amar AP, Mack WJ. Mechanical thrombectomy for acute ischemic stroke using the MERCI retriever and penumbra aspiration systems. *World Neurosurg.* 2011;6:S16-S23.

The ECASS studies 1 and 2:

Hacke W, Kaste M, Fieschi C, et al. Intravenous thrombolysis with recombinant tissue plasminogen activator for acute hemispheric stroke: the European Cooperative Acute Stroke Study (ECASS). *JAMA.* 1995;274:1017-1025.

Hacke W, Kaste M, Fieschi C, et al. Randomised double-blind placebo-controlled trial of thrombolytic therapy with intravenous alteplase in acute ischaemic stroke (ECASS II). *Lancet.* 1998;352:1245-1251.

Cardioembolic Stroke with Contraindications to Anticoagulation

A 74-year-old man with chronic atrial fibrillation was directed to discontinue warfarin therapy 3 months ago, when he was found to have significant iron-deficiency anemia with positive stool blood but negative endoscopic and radiologic workup of his GI tract. Last week, he had a transient left-visual-field loss, and this morning, about 8 hours ago, he had speech difficulty lasting approximately 45 minutes after getting out of the shower. In the remote past he had a left cerebellar stroke, which led to transient ataxia and vertigo, at which time the atrial fibrillation was discovered. On exam, there is some difficulty with naming, and fluency is reduced. Basic labs are normal. CT today reveals the old cerebellar stroke and a question of attenuation changes in the cortex near the left Sylvian fissure but is otherwise normal. Cardiac rate is irregular at approximately 76 beats per minute, BP is 134/76, and atrial fibrillation/flutter is identified on ECG. General exam is otherwise normal, as is neurological exam.

What do you do now?

The conclusion you will draw here is that this patient is very likely having recurrent cerebral ischemic events, probably occurring due to cardiac thromboemboli. Your next thought probably focuses on ways to halt this. Anticoagulation is appropriate, but there are real concerns here. First, the fact that this patient was felt to be a risk for serious gastrointestinal bleeding. Second, there is likely to be a new area of infarction, which can undergo hemorrhagic conversion, more likely if the patient is anticoagulated. It is too late to consider intravenous tPA so at least that decision is easy, although if the patient had been seen in an opportune time window, tPA might well have been a good option. So, it is time to make decisions about relative risks—the risks of anticoagulation, presumably with intravenous heparin, versus the risk of a new cardioembolic event. It is enormously difficult to use evidence to make these determinations because patients are unique in their risks for bleeding. In other words, no matter how applicable a randomized controlled double-blind study might seem for this patient, his unique features—most of which you do not know—will be paramount in terms of his risks of GI and cerebral hemorrhage with anticoagulation.

First, let's tackle the GI bleeding issue. Presumably, blood count is normal, and there is no active gastrointestinal bleeding. Stool can be checked for occult blood to confirm this. If all is well, short-term heparin therapy is probably safe. Long-term therapy with warfarin can be considered in a more leisurely fashion, perhaps after careful GI endoscopy. To increase comfort levels, hematocrit can be followed closely. There is considerable evidence that risk of recurrent stroke after initial event is highest over the next 2 weeks. It is a bit less certain how this breaks down over the next 2–3 days, but the risk is real and it is heartbreaking to have a patient re-stroke while recovering from the initial stroke. So, we have a positive vote for at least short-term anticoagulation.

What about the risk of converting a bland infarction into a hemorrhagic one? Evidence is controversial here, too. The size of the acute infarction is probably important, i.e. a large infarction is more likely to bleed. Avoiding very high spikes in blood pressure and carefully monitoring PTT will bias the odds against intracerebral hemorrhage. On the other hand, dropping BP in acute stroke can lead to extension of the infarctions, so the risks must be balanced. MRI (particularly DWI sequences) can help estimate the size of the stroke and can also detect even small amounts of bleeding early on, which would argue against heparin. But back to the original question: will the reduction in risk of recurrent infarction be outweighed by the risk of hemorrhagic conversion and resulting morbidity and mortality risks? It turns out that the risks tend to balance out pretty closely. Thus, evidence here is mixed.

Is there any advantage to using LMWH? No; in fact, there are disadvantages. The half-life of LMWH is long and it is inactivated by protamine to a much lesser extent. Therefore, if there is a bleeding complication, heparin is easier to reverse. Also, its activity is not assessable by PTT, so the degree of anticoagulation is generally inferred. And LMWH is expensive.

So what to do in terms of attempting to prevent recurrent cerebral ischemia in this patient? Evidence does not really help, so this becomes a clinical judgment problem. You are, however, not alone. This patient and his family can and should be enlisted to weigh the pros and cons. What they need to know is that the next stroke can be devastating, but that it is impossible to know when or if this will happen. Echocardiography can help by ruling out an intracardiac thrombus, but, of course, this is just a snapshot, and thrombi can begin to form at any time. The chances of recurrent stroke happening are generally below 5% in the first several days, so odds are good that this will not occur while they are weighing the options acutely. MRI can help by delineating the size of the stroke. Perhaps it is small but with a penumbra of impending ischemia, and therefore less likely to bleed than a large area of infarcted tissue. If the patient and family opt to avoid anticoagulation, this decision can be reassessed over the next few days. Cardiological consultation about acute and long-term plans for dealing with the atrial fibrillation with medication, cardioversion, or ablation therapy might help, but the success rate of these interventions has not been high enough to obviate the need for anticoagulation.

KEY POINTS TO REMEMBER

- Both systemic bleeding and intracerebral bleeding risks must be considered before starting anticoagulation in the acute post-stroke setting.
- When starting intravenous anticoagulation in the setting of acute cardioembolic stroke ("bridge therapy") the risks of hemorrhagic conversion of the infarction and reinfarction due to subsequent reembolization may be about equal.

- MRI of the brain and echocardiography can help the neurologist and patient assess pros and cons for starting heparin.
- If anticoagulation is begun in the acute post-stroke setting, strict control of BP, and close monitoring of bleeding parameters, are essential.

Further Reading

Hallevi H, Albright KC, Martin-Schild S, et al. Anticoagulation after cardioembolic stroke: to bridge or not to bridge? *Arch Neurol.* 2008;65:1169-1173.

Gladstone DJ, Bui E, Fang J, et al. Potentially preventable strokes in high-risk patients with atrial fibrillation who are not adequately anticoagulated. *Stroke.* 2009;40:235-240.

Jørgensen HS, Nakayama H, Reith J, Raaschou HO, Olsen TS. Acute stroke with atrial fibrillation: The Copenhagen Stroke Study. *Stroke.* 1996;27:1765-1769.

Singer OC, Humpich MC, Fiehler J, et al. . Risk for symptomatic intracerebral hemorrhage after thrombolysis assessed by DWI MRI. *Ann Neurol.* 2008;63:52-60.

Progressive Posterior Circulation Ischemia

A 68-year-old university professor is brought to the ED because of dysarthria that began near the end of his lecture about 6 hours ago. He continues to have difficulty speaking, but this seems to be improving. He also complains of some visual blurring on the left, which began on his way to the hospital. Last week he had some "clumsiness" in the right leg and arm for about 30 minutes. He has also had intermittent diplopia over the last several days. CT of the brain is normal other than some small white-matter low-signal regions and mild cortical atrophy. He has an indwelling cardiac pacemaker placed for bradycardia several years ago and cannot undergo MRI. He is on a beta blocker medication for hypertension but does not take it regularly due to side effects. He is also on a statin for hyperlipidemia, omeprazole for gastric reflux, and zolpidem for insomnia. General exam reveals BP of 158/98 and regular pulse of 78. Neck is supple. There is a bruit auscultated over the right carotid. Neurological exam reveals a mild facial droop on the right, some difficulty completely burying his left eye on left-lateral gaze, some mild right arm and leg weakness and patchy left homonymous hemianopsia. Coordination is normal. Gait is not tested due to the vertigo.

What do you do now?

This patient seems to have had a stuttering presentation of brainstem ischemia over the last several weeks. The posterior circulation is pretty clearly implicated due to the lack of cognitive symptoms, relative symmetry of face, arm and leg weakness, abducens palsy, and homonymous hemianopsia. The bilateral symptoms and lack of lower-brainstem dysfunction suggest basilar artery involvement and perhaps impending occlusion (BAO) with effects on primarily the ventral pons as well as territory supplied by the posterior cerebral artery on the right (left visual field deficit).

Basilar artery occlusion is one of the more potentially devastating conditions in neurology. It can present with TIAs involving brainstem and brain structures in the posterior fossa, as seen in this patient, with symptomatology including dysarthria, diplopia, hemiparesis, imbalance, loss of vision, sensory symptoms, and vertigo. Or BAO can present acutely with severe motor and brainstem symptoms along with impaired consciousness. It can lead, sometimes fairly quickly, to the locked-in syndrome. The most prominent risk factor for basilar thrombosis is hypertension, which this patient not only has but is not adequately treating.

Other possibilities for his presentation include a meningeal infectious or inflammatory process, vasculitis with multifocal ischemia, multifocal cardiogenic or paradoxical infarctions sparing anterior circulation, multiple CNS masses (e.g., neoplasm, abscesses), pontine hemorrhage, cerebellar infarction, hemorrhage with brainstem compression, or supratentorial mass or hemorrhage with herniation and subsequent brainstem compression. Preservation of consciousness and the normal CT tend to rule out most of these.

There are, at the moment, relatively mild-to-moderate symptoms; this presents an opportunity to intercede. More information must be obtained emergently in order to confirm our hypothesis and delineate the extent of the circulatory problem. Unfortunately, we cannot have the benefit of brainstem MRI imaging, but there are other options. The CT should be scrutinized to see whether there is a hyperdense basilar artery. CT arterial imaging of vertebrobasilar vessels should confirm our hypothesis, while at the same time providing some more important information on the anterior circulation, particularly regarding the bruit heard over the right carotid artery. Echocardiography can discover embolic sources in the heart and aorta. Transcranial Doppler can identify flow changes and thus occlusion in the basilar artery.

If BAO is seen, options remain even though the window of opportunity for intravenous tPA has closed. It is pretty clear that left untreated, many patients with BAO will have a poor outcome, so aggressive therapy may be appropriate. Unfortunately, there have been no randomized controlled trials of treatment in BAO. The choices are anticoagulation, intravenous tPA, intra-arterial tPA, and intra-arterial stenting or clot extraction or both. A large observational study looking at a number of patients with BAO who underwent one or more of these interventions unfortunately failed to support any one of the options over the others. In this basically healthy patient, any of these interventions might be sensible given that most symptoms have resolved, suggesting that significant brainstem infarction, with its risk of hemorrhage, has not happened yet. Intravenous heparinization is a quick approach but may not be effective. Intra-arterial thrombolysis with or without clot extraction and stenting seems most definitive and can also shed light on the nature of the occlusive disease. The problem is that CT or MR angiography should be done first, which may be time-consuming, and the clock is ticking. As always, whenever possible, the patient should be made aware of all these options, along with their potential benefits and risks, to enable him to participate fully in decision-making.

Blood pressure should be watched carefully. Unless thrombolysis is being considered, hypertension is not treated unless systolic exceeds 200 or diastolic exceeds 120. In potential thrombolysis situations, keeping systolic BP below 180 is probably wise. Sedating medication should be avoided since the patient's level of consciousness needs to be assessed frequently.

KEY POINTS TO REMEMBER

- Basilar thrombosis can present gradually with symptoms and signs referable to the pons and midbrain as well as occipital lobes.
- CT scanning is often nondiagnostic, but a hyperdense basilar artery can sometimes be seen.
- MRI, cerebrovascular imaging (MRA or CTA), echocardiography, and transcranial Doppler testing are all helpful in confirming the diagnosis and directing therapeutic decisions.
- Intravenous thrombolysis, intra-arterial thrombolysis, stenting, and thrombectomy are all possible interventions.

Further Reading

Goldmakher GV, Camargo EC, Furie KL, et al. Hyperdense basilar artery sign on unenhanced CT predicts thrombus and outcome in acute posterior circulation stroke. *Stroke*. 2009;40:134-139.

Muengtaweepongsa S, Singh NN, Cruz-Flores S. Pontine warning syndrome: case series and review of literature. *J Stroke Cerebrovasc Dis*. 2010;19:353-356.

Schonewille WJ, Wijman CA, Rueckert CM, et al. Treatment and outcomes of acute basilar artery occlusion in the Basilar Artery International Cooperation Study (BASICS). *Lancet Neurology*. 2009;8:724-730.

Recurring Transient Ischemic Attacks

A 73-year-old man was noted by his wife to slur his speech and complain of right-arm clumsiness earlier this evening. This resolved within minutes but seemed to reoccur several hours later and resolve quickly again. He is now in the ED and, despite an unwillingness to have medical care, admits that symptoms such as those he experienced today have bothered him in the past. He denies head pain, chest pain, and shortness of breath. Medical history is only remarkable for hypertension, which has been well controlled. He has no other neurological history. His general exam is normal except for his cataracts. Vital signs are normal, and there are no cardiac murmurs or carotid bruits. His neurological exam is normal. CT scan of the head is negative other than some mild cortical atrophy. He has made it clear that he intends to go home.

What do you do now?

This presentation is most likely the result of recurrent transient ischemia to the brain. The localization is probably the subcortical left frontal region, given that the arm and articulatory muscles seem most affected. Thus there is a suspicion of left middle cerebral artery (MCA) involvement. However, the lack of cognitive/dysphasic symptoms might suggest posterior circulation. Upper and lower limbs should be equally affected when pathological processes affect the corticospinal tract in the brainstem, but this rule is not entirely reliable. Could this presentation reflect nonischemic CNS dysfunction? Acephalgic migraine (migraine aura without headache) can occur in his age group, but very rarely in patients without a history of migraine. Partial seizures affecting the motor cortex can affect articulation and limb strength as well, so this is another possibility. However, migraine auras and partial seizures are generally manifested by "positive phenomena." In the case of migraine, by paresthesias, visual images, and scotomata; in the case of partial motor seizures, by dystonic or clonic activity, rather than weakness. Of course, there is always the possibility of partial seizures not noted by observers, with subsequent Todd's paralysis mimicking a TIA. Another possibility is so-called "re-expression" of symptoms from an old stroke on the basis of metabolic or hypoperfusion conditions. In the case above, the CT tends to rule this out. (Interestingly, diagnosis of TIA is not easy, even for stroke specialists, a group of whom were found in a recent study to differ in conclusions about the same cases.)

If this patient's recurrent symptoms do indeed stem from ischemia, what are the possible etiologies? Cardiogenic or artery-to-artery embolization is certainly possible, but the stereotypic manifestations in this patient are rather convincing for small-vessel stenosis. A workup to rule out other causes is worth doing quickly, however, including MRI of the brain to look for old or more recent stroke, and MRA to see if either large-vessel (carotid, vertebral, basilar) or smaller vessel stenosis is present. Transcranial Doppler aimed at identifying flow changes in the MCA can be a useful addition. CT angiography may be more sensitive than MRA for assessing the caliber of intracranial arteries. Echocardiography is worthwhile not only to evaluate for intracardiac thrombus, valvular disease, and patent foramen ovale, but also to check the efficiency of the heart, in case reduced cardiac outflow might be contributory to this patient's symptoms. Hypercoagulability will also need to be ruled out with CBC and clotting factor testing. General metabolic status will need to be determined as well as ESR. Giant-cell arteritis does not affect intracranial vessels, but extradural vertebral artery involvement has been described. If all of these tests are negative, consideration should be given to conventional intra-arterial angiography to search for focal stenosis. Cerebral arteritides, while generally multifocal, can (rarely) lead to stereotypic TIA-like episodes.

If a focally stenotic MCA or MCA branch consistent with this patient's symptomatology is identified, treatment must focus on management of hypertension and any other possible risk factors, including statin treatment of hyperlipidemia. In the short term, however, maintenance of adequate blood pressure may be the most helpful intervention aimed at preventing permanent ischemic damage to the territory supplied by the focally stenotic artery. This quandary is usually approached carefully by allowing BP to remain on the higher side, as long as it does not exceed 220 mm, at least until symptoms have disappeared. Antithrombotic therapy with oral aspirin (325 mg daily) plus clopidogrel and rouvastatin is standard therapy for symptomatic intracranial arterial stenosis. Interestingly, more aggressive antithrombotic therapy with warfarin has not proven any better than aspirin so should not be used initially. On the other hand, if patients like this one continue to experience symptoms despite modification of risk factors and aspirin/clopidogrel therapy, using warfarin instead may be appropriate. For focal intracranial large artery stenosis, endovascular stenting procedures are being studied but none are supported by evidence.

KEY POINTS TO REMEMBER

- Recurrent transient neurological symptoms are best regarded as a warning for impending cerebral ischemic damage unless proven otherwise.
- Cerebral ischemia tends to produce "negative phenomena," whereas migraine and focal epilepsy produce more "positive symptomatology."
- TIAs should warrant a search for the contributing arterial causes as well as risk factors for stroke.
- MRA, CTA, transcranial Doppler, and conventional angiography can all supply important information about arteriopathy in cases of TIA and stroke.

Further Reading

Castel J, Mlynash M, Lee K, et al. Agreement regarding diagnosis of transient ischemic attack fairly low among stroke-trained neurologists. *Stroke.* 2010;41:1367-1370.

Chimowitz MI, Lynn MJ, Howlett-Smith H, et al. Comparison of warfarin and aspirin for symptomatic intracranial arterial stenosis. *NEJM.* 2005;352:1305-1316.

Easton JD, Saver JL, Albers GW, et al. Definition and evaluation of transient ischemic attack: a scientific statement for healthcare professionals from the American Heart Association/American Stroke Association Stroke Council; Council on Cardiovascular Surgery and Anesthesia; Council on Cardiovascular Radiology and Intervention; Council on Cardiovascular Nursing; and the Interdisciplinary Council on Peripheral Vascular Disease. *Stroke.* 2009;40:2276-2293.

Kasner SE, Lynn MJ, Chimowitz MI, et al. Warfarin v. aspirin for symptomatic intracranial arterial stenosis: subgroup analysis from WASID. *Neurology.* 2006;67:1275-1278.

17 Intractable Status Epilepticus

A 28-year-old man with reported lifelong history of epilepsy previously treated with multiple medications is brought to the ED by his girlfriend, who tells the staff that he has been seizure-free and healthy for months but stopped taking his most recent medications, levatiracetam and clonazepam, last week. The generalized motor seizures he began having 2 hours ago have been occurring nearly continuously. She tells you he is seriously allergic to phenytoin. His vital signs are normal, ECG is normal, neck is supple between seizures, but he only arouses minimally between convulsions. Lorazepam has been given twice at a dose of 2 mg each time with little effect.

What do you do now?

Status epilepticus (SE) is defined as "more than 30 minutes of continuous seizure activity or two or more sequential seizures without full recovery of consciousness between seizures" (Epilepsy Foundation). It is a neurological emergency because of the understanding that irreversible brain changes can occur as a result (the hippocampus seems to be particularly sensitive), and the sooner seizure activity can be halted the better the prognosis. General support must include close scrutiny of respiration, support of BP or perhaps reduction when BP rises precipitously, and monitoring of temperature. Many patients in SE can become hyperthermic, which must be addressed. Acidosis usually occurs but resolves with termination of the seizure and usually is not treated. Cardiac arrhythmias can also occur.

The most common cause of SE is discontinuation of medications, but new exacerbating factors must always be ruled out. Therefore, it is important to search for infection including meningitis or encephalitis, metabolic derangements (sodium, calcium, hepatic and renal dysfunction), drug toxicity (cocaine, amphetamines), ethanol or barbiturate withdrawal, new stroke, intracranial mass lesion, subarachnoid hemorrhage, and sequelae of head trauma, such as subdural hematomata. Initial workup is done simultaneously with administration of anticonvulsants and should generally include electrolytes, glucose, BUN, creatinine, liver enzymes, blood count, drug screen, urinalysis, CT of the head, and LP if there is any suspicion of meningitis, encephalitis, or subarachnoid hemorrhage.

As treatment of the seizures begins, it is important to make sure the patient is safe, to ensure airway patency, and to give the patient glucose, thiamine, and possibly naloxone. Lorazepam (0.1 mg/kg) IV over 5 minutes can be tried even if benzodiazepines have been attempted. If this is not quickly helpful, fosphenytoin or phenytoin is generally given. If available, fosphenytoin is a better choice because it can be given faster and does not carry the risk of "purple-glove syndrome" as phenytoin does. (An approach to addressing SE is summarized in Table 17.1.)

The dose of fosphenytoin is 15 to 20 mg phenytoin equivalents/kg. However, this patient is said to be allergic to phenytoin, so this is not an option. An alternative is to load with valproate intravenously with a dose of 20 to 30 mg/kg over 5 minutes.

If seizures continue, the next step is generally phenobarbital given 20 mg/kg IV at a rate of approximately 50–100 mg per minute. However,

TABLE 17.1   **An Approach to Status Epilepticus**

1	Ensure airway, respiration, and circulation. Start IV with normal saline Oxygen + Glucose + Thiamine
2	Lorazepam 0.1 mg per kg by IV push, but less than 2 mg/min Bedside EEG running if possible
3	Phenytoin 20 mg/kg at 50 mg/min or Fosphenytoin 15 to 20 mg "Phenytoin Equivalents" loading dose at a maximum rate of 150 mg "Phenytoin Equivalents" per minute
4	Intubate; Phenobarbital 20 mg/kg to maximum 100 mg/min or Pentobarbital 5 to 15 mg/kg, slowly, following EEG, to suppress all epileptiform activity. Continue 0.5 to 5 mg/kg per hour to maintain EEG suppression. Or Propofol IV drip

before this is done serious consideration should be given to elective intubation since the addition of phenobarbital in a patient already treated with benzodiazepines may lead to ventilatory failure, particularly in patients with any pulmonary disease or in elderly patients who may have slower clearance of the benzodiazepines. Another choice here is levatiracetam, which is an attractive idea because the patient was previously taking this medication with good results. Loading dose should be 50 mg/kg IV and can be given relatively rapidly. Lacosamide,a new antiepileptic drug available in IV form, might be effective in refractory SE but evidence is lacking at present.

If seizures continue, the next step will need to be into the realm of general anesthesia with medications such as propofol, midazolam, or pentobarbital via IV drip. These are generally given by the anesthesiology team, with a loading dose followed by continuous IV drip. A simplified streamlined approach might consist of (1) lorazepam up to 8 mg IV, (2) loading dose of phosphenytoin, then (3) propofol.

Bedside EEG monitoring is enormously helpful from the very first step, and if available should be instituted as soon as possible. Its main purpose is to ensure that subclinical seizures are not occurring. When general anesthesia is administered, the goal is to produce a burst-suppression pattern on EEG.

- Status epilepticus is diagnosed when seizure activity continues for more than 30 minutes or when a patient is experiencing repetitive seizures for more than 30 minutes without regaining full consciousness between them.
- Control of seizures must be achieved as quickly as possible, concurrent with a search for causes including meningitis, stroke, drug intoxication, metabolic derangements, or head trauma.
- The general order of medication choices consists of benzodiazepines, phenytoin, phenobarbital, and general anesthesia.
- General medical monitoring for hyperthermia, hypertension, hypoxia, renal dysfunction, electrolyte imbalance, and arrhythmia must occur simultaneously with treatment of SE.

Further Reading

Hirsch LJ. The status of intravenous valproate for status. *Epilepsy Curr*. 2007;7:96-98.

Knake S, Gruener J, Hattemer K, et al. Intravenous levetiracetam in the treatment of benzodiazepine refractory status epilepticus. *J Neurol Neurosurg Psychiatry*. 2008;795:588-589.

Ramael S, Daoust A, Otoul C, et al. Levetiracetam intravenous infusion: a randomized, placebo-controlled safety and pharmacokinetic study. *Epilepsia*. 2006;47:1128-1135.

Treiman DM, Meyers PD, Walton NY, et al. A comparison of four treatments for generalized convulsive status epilepticus. Veterans Affairs Status Epilepticus Cooperative Study Group. *N Engl J Med*. 1998;339:792-798.

18 Severe Intractable Headache

A 38-year-old known migraineur is being seen in the ED for a severe headache that has failed to respond to ketorolac 60 mg IM, prochlorperazine 25 mg IM, and lorazepam 4 mg IM. She tried sumatriptan perorally (PO) at home last night, which was ineffective. She states that the pain is unbearable and beseeches you to "just give me a shot of morphine—That helped last time!" You see that her last ED visit for headache occurred 2 weeks ago and that she has had 9 visits to the ED in the last 6 months. She also complains of some nausea, severe photo- and phonophobia, and some mild vertigo. She is taking amitriptyline 100 mg qhs, sumatriptan 100 mg ("when my insurance company will let me have some"), topiramate 100 mg bid, propranolol (long-acting) 80 mg bid, and clonazepam 2 mg qhs. She also takes hydrocodone and butalbital, as well as an assortment of over-the-counter analgesics, regularly. She has no abnormal neurological findings on exam. Vital signs are normal and neck is supple. CT of the head is normal.

What do you do now?

There is no emergency room physician who cannot recall many patients with a nearly identical presentation. The headache is most likely migraine but making sure to rule out secondary causes of headaches is important— intracranial mass, hemorrhage, meningoencephalitis, hydrocephalus, or abscess are all highly unlikely with a normal exam. But cervical arterial dissection, vasculitis, reversible cerebral vasoconstriction syndrome, toxicity or metabolic derangement, cerebral venous thrombosis, and an array of less-common causes of headache must be considered. A way to decide quickly whether to embark on a workup for these is to ask the following questions:

- Was the headache onset sudden ("thunderclap")?
- Is this either a new headache or a change from a preexisting headache pattern?
- Is there fever, significant hypertension, or neck stiffness?
- Are there any findings on neurological exam, including cognitive dysfunction?
- Is this headache occurring in the setting of systemic illness (e.g., acquired immune deficiency syndrome (AIDS) or cancer)?

Generally, the answer to all of these is "No." But if any of these "red flags" are present, imaging of the head, lumbar puncture, cerebrovascular imaging, and extensive metabolic screening may be indicated.

If this is indeed simply another migraine, why is it so unresponsive to medication, and why is she having to come to the ED so often despite prophylactic medication and appropriate acute headache medication? Unfortunately, the medications are most likely a large part of this patient's problems. When migraine patients overuse analgesic and/or migraine abortive medications, headache frequency increases via an as yet poorly understood mechanism. Previously termed "analgesic rebound," this condition is referred to as Medication Overuse Headache (MOH), and it is very challenging to treat. First, patients in this state tend not to respond to acute treatments, even those that were once useful. Second, when patients attempt to discontinue offending medications, such as butalbital, triptans, and mixed analgesics (all of which this patient is using), headaches worsen further, pushing them to actually increase analgesic medications. Finally, prophylactic medications become ineffective as well. The frequency and doses of the analgesic/abortive medications needed to produce this syndrome probably varies from patient to patient, and with different acute medications, but usage on 3 days per week or more is generally enough to cause MOH.

So, an apparently unsolvable problem confronts the medical team here. Fortunately, there are some reasonably good options for immediate control of pain that will not escalate the problem of medication overuse. Ketorolac was a good choice but was not effective, possibly because of the frequent use of over-the-counter medications in the nonsteroidal anti-inflammatory drug (NSAID) category. Another option is intravenous valproate, which is given as a 500 to 1000 mg bolus. Intravenous magnesium sulfate is another option and is given in doses of 1 g up to 5 g total as slow IV push. Intravenous dihydroergotamine (DHE) at a dose of 1 mg is another option, although it should not be given in close temporal proximity to a triptan. Occipital nerve blocks seem to be very helpful for some patients, though the mechanism is not well understood. Intravenous neuroleptic medication can be extremely useful for acute refractory migraine. A good choice is prochlorperazine 10 mg. Because of the risk of dystonia, this is often administered with diphenhydramine 25 mg intravenously. Finally, parenteral corticosteroids, either as a one-time dose or followed by a tapering dose over several days. A typical initial dose might be 6 to 8 mg of dexamethasone.

Opioids are to be avoided. While they can certainly relieve pain, the effect is temporary, and large doses are generally required, leading to significant sedation. Plus, opioids will just amplify the medication overuse condition. Patients who have had opioid treatment in the past may remember the gratifying relief of pain (and perhaps euphoria) and ask for it again. Although this is interpreted as illicit drug-seeking, it might better be framed as appropriate protective behavior. Nonetheless, the request for opioids is to be countered with clear explanations of why they are not indicated. If all approaches fail, the patient can be admitted and treated more aggressively, perhaps with a course of intravenous DHE infusions or parenteral neuroleptics.

Some or all of the above are usually successful in alleviating the patient's headache, or at least significantly reducing its severity. But the problem of headache recurrence, very likely in the setting of medication overuse, remains. Patients such as this one must be enlisted in the fight to limit acute pain medications and it may be reasonable to refer them to a headache specialist, who can simplify and adjust the prophylactic program and help to design a multimodal treatment plan.

- Even patients with a known headache disorder must be thoughtfully evaluated for the presence of a new secondary cause when presenting to the emergency department with intractable pain.
- There are a number of parenteral pharmacological choices for acute migraine treatment, including ketorolac, dihydroergotamine, magnesium, valproate, neuroleptics, and corticosteroids.
- Occipital nerve blocks may be a useful addition to the treatment options.
- Medication overuse may complicate the picture of acute refractory migraine and must be addressed.

Further Reading

Friedman BW. Review: Phenothiazines relieve acute migraine headaches in the ED and are better than other active agents for some outcomes. *Ann Intern Med.* 2010;152:JC4-JC11.

Katsarava Z, Holle D, Diener H-C. Medication overuse headache. *Curr Neurol Neurosci Rep.* 2009;9:115-119.

Mauskop A. Acute treatment of migraine headaches. *Seminars in Pain Medicine.* 2004;2:72-75.

Silberstein SD, Freitag FG, and Bigal ME. Migraine treatment. In: Silberstein SD, Lipton RB, and Dalessio DJ. *Wolff's Headache and other Head Pain.* 8th ed. New York: Oxford University Press; 2008: 153-176.

19 Acute Lumbar Radiculopathy

A 64-year-old dentist became aware of pain in his right lateral thigh and leg after arising this morning. He played in a long tennis match yesterday. Pain can be aching or lancinating, and he admits to intermittent aching pain in his right buttock for about a year. Pain has become intolerable over the past 3-4 hours and he is close to tears. He tried 800 mg of ibuprofen, which was completely ineffective. He denies chest pain, back pain, and any pain in the left leg. On exam he is unable to move his torso in the anteroposterior or side-to-side direction. He has a diminished ankle-jerk reflex on the right, and there is some weakness on standing on his right toes. Straight-leg-raising is moderately positive on the right. Perirectal sensation is good, and anal wink is present. Plain x-rays of his spine reveal osteophytes throughout the lumbar and upper sacral region but no sign of fracture or inflammation.

What do you do now?

This patient presents with an extremely common condition, but one which can present at very different levels of severity. There are several questions to answer in these cases and once this is done, the therapeutic direction is usually pretty easy to determine.

Question number one: Is this truly a radicular pattern of pain? It certainly seems to be radicular, involving the right S1 root. Hip pathology and even vascular disease in the leg can cause unusual pain radiation patterns, but here the location of the pain is classic for S1 radiculopathy, there is reflex change involving S1 innervated muscles, and there is some paresis in an S1 innervated muscle (gastrocnemius). Lumbar strain in muscles or ligaments, which might be suggested by his exertions the day before, is unlikely to be the sole cause given that there are clearly neuropathic components. Cauda equina region involvement by large disc, infection, or neoplasm is not suggested by any symptoms relating to multiple bilateral roots, urinary incontinence, or saddle anesthesia.

The most common causes for lumbosacral root pain are herniated disc and lumbosacral spinal stenosis due to arthritis. Infection, or neoplastic involvement of a lumbosacral root is possible but rare, and the plain films rule out invasive/destructive neoplasm or significant osteomyelitis. The two most commonly involved nerves are L5, which leads to foot-drop and pain radiating to the large toe, and S1, which is manifested by lateral leg pain, decreased plantar flexion strength, and reduced or absent ankle jerk.

Question number two: Is there any weakness? It is always hard to judge motor power in a limb that is painful. And moderate weakness is sometimes undetectable via manual motor testing. However, the examiner of this patient tells us that a *functional* test of strength—walking on tiptoes—is abnormal on the symptomatic side. This, of course, might be related to exacerbation of pain in that position, but one would assume other muscles would be somewhat affected, and they are strong. A helpful objective clue, and one that suggests the pathology here, is the absence of the ankle-jerk reflex on the symptomatic side.

The presence of weakness should raise concern that the disease process has already caused some disability and that an expeditious workup and initiation of treatment is indicated.

Question number three: Can pain be adequately controlled while physical methods are used to assist the healing process? This patient is in severe pain, but it should be responsive to oral or parenteral pain medication. There is always the concern that opioid medication is being sought for euphoric properties and that this can lead to addiction if not carefully controlled. This is a valid concern, but if this patient's history is not notable for previous abuse of prescription medication, it is likely he is a good candidate for short-term opioid medication.

So, now what? You can control the pain temporarily, but exam suggests that measures should be taken to at least attempt to halt the process of root compression. In this patient's age group, spinal stenosis is more likely than acute herniated disc. What may have happened is that the exertion of the day before caused right S1 trauma due to stretching of the root across a very narrow foramen. Interestingly, lost reflexes and strength loss are sometimes reversible, so therapeutic intervention is wise. The majority of patients will, in fact, improve without surgical intervention, although it is difficult to predict the chances for any individual patient. Physical therapeutic approaches tend to be the usual choice, but there have been no real studies of these manual therapies for acute lumbosacral radiculopathy. And styles of therapy tend to differ fairly significantly, with disciples of various approaches each using a "one-size-fits-all" approach.

Systemic corticosteroids may be appropriate, but here again there is very little evidence to support this, or good guidelines for choice of medication or dose. Epidural injection of steroids is likewise poorly supported, although there are a number of case series suggesting significant benefit.

Surgery for acute lumbosacral radicular pain depends on the cause of the pain. MRI of the spine can be very helpful here in distinguishing nerve compression by a ruptured disc from pain due to severe foraminal encroachment. If it is due to an acute herniated disc, surgery is done to remove part or all of the disc. In spinal-stenosis-induced pain, surgery attempts to enlarge foramina via laminectomies, which may need to be stabilized by hardware inserted into the spine. While no controlled studies have been done that confirm the benefits of surgery, a number of comparative studies seem to show superiority of surgery over nonsurgical management for up to 2 years. After this end point, outcomes seem equivalent. Nonsurgical approaches also include weight loss for any patients who are overweight, avoidance of load bearing, and only nonexacerbating exercise.

- Acute lumbosacral radicular pain is usually due to disc rupture and herniation or exacerbation of spinal stenosis, but neoplasm, fracture, infection, and compressive cauda equine syndrome must be excluded.
- The most common lumbosacral roots to be symptomatic are S1 and L5, although L4 can also be involved.
- Pain can usually be controlled medically.
- Manual and surgical approaches to acute radicular pain seem to be equivalent in terms of long-term outcome, although surgical intervention can provide some additional benefit in the short term.

Further Reading

Cuckler JM, Bernini PA, Wiesel SW, Booth RE Jr, Rothman RH, Pickens GT. The use of epidural steroids in the treatment of lumbar radicular pain. A prospective, randomized, double-blind study. *J Bone Joint Surg Am.* 1985;67:63-66.

Holve RL, Barkan H. Oral steroids in initial treatment of acute sciatica. *J Am Board Fam Med.* 2008;21:469-474.

Pengel LHM, Herbert RD, Maher CG, Refshauge KM. Acute low back pain: systematic review of its prognosis. *BMJ.* 2003;327:323-330.

20 Post-traumatic Paraplegia

A 27-year-old was skiing on an icy snow hill, lost
control and fell, sliding approximately 50 feet. He was
immobilized and carried off the hill by bystanders and
then brought to the ED via helicopter, where he was
found to have a right-clavicular fracture as well as a
fracture of his jaw. He cannot move his legs. Exam was
remarkable for an absence of spontaneous movement
in the lower extremities. Reflexes are diminished in the
legs and tone is somewhat flaccid. Sensation seems to
be diminished in the legs as well, but he states he feels
some sensation. Anal wink is preserved. Abdominal
reflexes are not appreciated. The remainder of the exam
is normal.

What do you do now?

The results of a spinal cord injury can be divided into *primary* and *secondary* injury. Primary injury refers to the damage induced by stretching or other deforming injuries of the spinal cord, penetrating trauma to the spinal cord, and/or compression of the spinal cord by fracture fragments or hematomas. Secondary injury refers to damage incurred as a result of cord edema, hemorrhage, and infarction of the cord, which occurs in the hours to days following the primary injury. The primary damage is often irreversible, and immediate post-traumatic care is directed at reducing the potential for secondary damage to the spinal cord. In the field, patients are immobilized; airway, breathing, and circulatory functions are ensured; and speedy transport to a spine injury center is expedited. The neurologist's role in the ED is generally to identify the site of lesions and to help discover various pathologies, including disk herniation, hematomas, fractures, etc. Plain films of the spine should be done, along with pelvic and long-bone films if there is any suspicion of trauma there. MRI is ideal for identifying compression by disc or blood. CT is better for revealing bony architecture, including fractures.

This patient seems to have suffered a thoracic cord injury. It is considered to be incomplete because there is some sacral root sparing, as well as some preservation of sensation in the legs. The level is unclear because the patient is vague about sensory level. The absence of abdominal reflexes (governed by T9 and T11 roots in most cases) suggests a lesion above T9 and this could be even higher, even low cervical as compression of the cord extrinsically may preferentially affect the corticospinal fibers involving leg function first. (Cervical-spinal-cord traumatic injuries are by far the most common due to the lower spine being relatively fixed). In this case, there seems to be an element of spinal shock— with decreased reflexes and tone in the lower extremities. This can persist for several days, eventually leading to the more typical upper motor neuron injury pattern of hyper-reflexia and spasticity. This case may also represent a process involving multiple roots in the cauda equina, hence the need for imaging.

Certain spinal syndromes are worth knowing well so that imaging and exam findings can be well understood. In some fortunate cases, patients will have suffered what is known as *spinal cord concussion*, which implies a more or less lack of permanent anatomic damage to the cord. There may be transient flaccid paralysis, but good recovery occurs relatively quickly. Alternatively, *spinal cord contusion* may have occurred, causing cord edema and perhaps petechial hemorrhages, resulting ultimately in some neurological residual deficits.

Spinal cord transection, of course, implies permanent damage to the cord. The *anterior spinal cord syndrome* manifests with paralysis and loss of pain sensation below the level of spinal injury, with preservation of touch, vibratory, and position sensation. The *central spinal cord syndrome* produces motor and sensory deficits, which are greater in the upper extremities if the trauma resulted in damage to the cervical cord. This is often the result of cervical hyperextension injuries. The *Brown-Sequard syndrome* is seen after damage to one side of the spinal cord and includes ipsilateral paresis, proprioception and vibratory loss below the level of injury, and contralateral pain and temperature loss below injury level. This is a pattern seen after penetrating injury.

Initial treatment of traumatic spinal cord injury usually includes the administration of methylprednisolone in the first 8 hours despite some controversy about the evidence for its efficacy. The dose is 30 mg/kg given intravenously over 15 minutes followed later by a lower dose of 5.4 mg/kg infusion over the next 23 hours, and longer if treatment was delayed more than 3–4 hours. Gangliosides (usually GM-1) and antioxidants given early have been recommended by some despite limited evidence to support their use. Surgical intervention in these cases does not generally improve the primary injury to the spinal cord, but if there is compression from any bony or disc material or blood, evacuation and stabilization of the spinal cord is essential, and is probably best done as quickly as is safe for the patient.

KEY POINTS TO REMEMBER

- After spinal injury, patients must be immobilized in the field; airway, breathing, and circulation ensured; and then brought to a spinal trauma center as soon as possible.
- Determination of other injuries and localization of the site(s) of damage must be done quickly.
- Imaging is done to visualize bones, discs, and hemorrhage—MRI is best for most issues, but CT is more accurate regarding bony pathology.
- Treatment of spinal cord injury with intravenous methylprednisolone is standard practice in most centers, but evidence is mixed for its efficacy.
- In order to prevent secondary spinal cord injury, surgical decompression is done when there is compression of the spinal cord.

Further Reading

Bracken MB, Shepard MJ, Holford TR, et al. Administration of methylprednisolone for 24 or 48 hours or tirilazad mesylate for 48 hours in the treatment of acute spinal cord injury. Results of the Third National Acute Spinal Cord Injury Study. *JAMA*. 1997;277:1597–1604.

Geisler FH, Dorsey FC, Coleman WP. Recovery of motor function after spinal-cord injury—a randomized, placebo controlled trial with GM-1 ganglioside. *N Engl J Med*. 1991;324:1829–1838.

Qi Chen, Feng Li, Zhong Fang, et al. Timing of surgical decompression for acute traumatic cervical spinal cord injury. *Neurosurg Q*. 2012;22:61–68.

Acute Severe Facial Pain

An 84-year-old woman is seen in the ED for excruciating
right-facial pain, which has been bothering her for
the past several weeks and escalated this morning.
The most painful territory is in the right preauricular
and lower cheek areas, and she is in tears due to its
severity and incessancy. The pain feels "electrical" and
"burning." She denies headache or pain anywhere else,
changes in vision, weakness and imbalance. She recalls
no rashes or other recent illnesses. CT scan of the
head is normal as is routine hematology and chemistry
blood testing. Neurological exam is remarkable only
for some hearing loss bilaterally, and reduction in
reflexes diffusely. She will not let you touch her face as
it exacerbates the pain, but there is no tenderness over
the mastoid or areas outside the painful region. There
are no skin changes noted.

What do you do now?

This patient probably has a classic case of trigeminal neuralgia (TN), which can become intractable. Pain can mount to such an extent that some patients become suicidal. Fortunately, there are some useful strategies to address pain both acutely and long-term, but first, steps should be taken to completely rule out other causes of the pain.

TN is considered a "primary neuralgia," meaning it has no underlying cause. This is, of course, not true, because it probably results from some as yet unknown insult to the trigeminal nerve or nucleus. Many believe TN to be the result of compression of the proximal trigeminal nerve by an artery, often the superior cerebellar artery. At any rate, it is your responsibility to exclude other causes. Meningeal inflammatory/infectious processes, tumors, aneurysms, and abscesses can cause irritation of the trigeminal nerve; and a multiple sclerosis (MS) plaque near the root-entry zone in the pons can also produce secondary trigeminal neuralgic syndromes. Herpetic infection of the nerve, as well as post-herpetic neuralgia, can be the cause. Inflammatory, infectious, thrombotic, granulomatous, neoplastic, and vascular lesions in the cavernous sinus can also cause a TN picture. In these cases, only the first 2 divisions of the trigeminal are involved at most, because the third division, the mandibular branch, does not pass through the cavernous sinus. Cluster headache, paroxysmal hemicrania (PH), and the syndrome of "short-lasting unilateral neuralgiform headache with conjunctival injection and tearing" (SUNCT) can all lead to pain that can be mistaken for TN. Cluster headaches are generally much longer than the lancinations of TN. PH and SUNCT are shorter, but all three of these primary headache disorders are associated with autonomic features such as tearing and nasal congestion ipsilateral to the pain, which are not present in the case above. Infection or neoplastic disease in the sinus, orbit, ear, or mouth can also mimic TN (Table 21.1).

A good workup for suspected TN then would include brain MRI, with and without contrast, to exclude MS, brainstem region masses or infection, and cavernous-sinus-region lesions. Lumbar puncture might be indicated, particularly if there are other cranial nerves involved, to rule out a meningeal infectious or inflammatory process such as sarcoidosis or Lyme disease. A search for herpetic lesions or scars might be revealing. And a very good head and neck exam should be done to exclude an otic, orbital, or sinus lesion.

TABLE 21.1 **Differential Diagnosis of Trigeminal Neuralgia**

Cavernous Sinus syndromes

Cluster headache

Paroxysmal hemicranias

SUNCT (Short-lasting Unilateral Neuralgiform headache attacks with Conjunctival injection and Tearing)

Hemifacial spasm

Migraine headache

Multiple sclerosis

Post-herpetic neuralgia

Subarachnoid hemorrhage

Sinus, ocular, or otic pathology

Herpetic and post-herpetic neuralgia

Most patients with TN can get good long-lasting pain relief with judicious use of antineuralgia medication such as carbamazepine (400–800 mg daily given in the long-acting form bid), gabapentin, amitriptyline, or baclofen, as well as a number of second-line prophylactic medications. However, the problem confronting you now is how to stop her acute pain. Intravenous phenytoin has been helpful for a number of patients at a dose of 15 mg/kg infused slowly. Fosphenytoin is safer and can be infused more rapidly. Occipital nerve blocks have helped some patients with acute pain. Other parenteral anticonvulsants have been tried, including levetiracetam. Neuroleptic antiemetics have also been helpful for selected patients in excruciating pain from TN. Chlorpromazine, for example, at a dose of 25–50 mg IV given carefully with dimenhydramine seems to be effective in acute exacerbations of TN. This can be very sedating so patients must be watched carefully after administration.

TN typically produces lancinating pain and can be triggered by touch, as in this patient. The usual areas of pain fall into the maxillary and mandibular regions of the face (served by the lower two divisions of the trigeminal nerve). Patients may be seen to have contractions of their face on the side of pain (hence the synonym for TN—"tic dolouroux"). This is not to be confused with hemifacial spasm, thought to be due to irritation of the facial nerve. Some patients, however, complain of more aching type pain without the other features of TN. This has been termed "Atypical Facial Pain" and carries the connotation of psychogenic etiology. It seems much more likely that it is simply a different manifestation of the same process—trigeminal irritation, and the search for secondary causes and successful treatment is very similar.

KEY POINTS TO REMEMBER

- Acute exacerbations of TN can be excruciating and can even lead to suicidality.
- Prophylactic pharmacological treatment of TN is generally very effective.
- There are several options for acute treatment of TN exacerbations, although clear evidence of their efficacy is not yet available.
- Atypical Facial Pain is a somewhat pejorative term that probably represents an overlap syndrome with many features of TN.

Further Reading

Cheshire WP Jr. The shocking tooth about trigeminal neuralgia. *N Engl J Med.* 2000;342:2003.

Cruccu G, Gronseth G, Alksne J, et al. AAN-EFNS guidelines on trigeminal neuralgia management. *Eur J Neurol.* 2008;15:1013-1028.

Gazzeri R. Atypical trigeminal neuralgia associated with tongue piercing. *JAMA.* 2006;296:1836-1842.

Tate R, Rubin LM, Krajewski KC. Treatment of refractory trigeminal neuralgia with intravenous phenytoin. *Am J Health Syst Pharm.* 2011;68:2059-2061.

PART III

Neuropsychiatric, Ethical, and Legal Dilemmas

22 Neurological Patients and Decision-making Capacity

A disheveled elderly man is brought to the ED after having a witnessed generalized convulsion. He is awake and interactive but argumentative and insisting upon leaving the ED. He smells of alcohol and has a temperature of 102° F. His neck is a bit stiff in the anteroposterior direction and rhonchi are heard bilaterally on auscultation of his lungs. Electrolytes are normal but WBC count is 17,000 with immature forms seen. Neurological exam reveals intact cranial nerves and a grossly normal symmetrical motor and sensory examination. Gait seems unsteady with a wide base. Chest x-ray reveals bilateral infiltrates and a small pleural effusion on the right. CT scan of the head done soon after admission to the ED reveals cortical atrophy and ventriculomegaly (hydrocephalus ex vacuo), but is otherwise normal. He refused to have an LP.

What do you do now?

When patients seem to make irrational medical decisions, the issue arises as to whether or not they have the capacity to make these important decisions. Or, in legal terms, whether they are "competent" in this area. A good way to approach this determination is to try to answer the following questions:

- Does he appreciate the medical situation and the potential consequences of his decisions regarding recommendations made by the medical team?
- Is he able to communicate his choices to you?
- Is his decision stable over several conversations, rather than impulsive and variable?
- Is his decision consistent with his values and health goals?

These questions are sometimes not easy to answer, so help must be sought from family members, close friends, and your psychology and psychiatry associates. Patients in delirium or coma clearly lack decision-making capacity, as do severely demented patients. But the difficulty mounts when dealing with patients exhibiting milder deficits for which there may be no clear tests, without resorting to lengthy neuropsychological assessments. One tool was developed, the MacArthur Competence Assessment Test, with psychiatric patients in mind. It consists of three spheres of assessment—understanding, reasoning, and appreciation. It has been studied for a number of years and seems to be a good indicator, but with an agitated patient such as this it may not be a useful option. The best approach, of course, is to build rapport with the patient, enlist the aid of his family or friends, and begin to collaborate about the best course of action. Often, a bit of reassurance, demonstration of full support for the patient's rights, and patience will result in a comfortable patient who trusts you and the medical team enough to accept your advice. Sometimes, an ideal way to achieve this is to present the patient with a choice or series of choices along different, but all reasonable, diagnostic and/or treatment paths. This prevents the patient from feeling backed into a corner and having to say yes or no. Instead he can choose the option that fits his own preferences. During this process you should also make sure *you* are communicating your recommendations well and fairly.

If despite all you do, the patient remains intransigent, you have to step back (literally—and sometimes into another room or area entirely) and ask yourself if the patient's decision will put his life at risk or likely lead to irreversible harm to himself. If not, and you cannot prove him to be lacking decision-making capacity, you probably have to respect his wishes. However, if there is grave danger, a legal precedent called the "emergency exception" gives physicians the leeway to go ahead with treatment in a life-threatening situation (or one that will lead to serious disability in the absence of treatment). In the case above, this emergency exception probably applies. The clock is ticking on a possible case of bacterial meningitis, testing is not particularly invasive, and there is no family member to consult, much less the patient's durable power of attorney for health care. Of course, if this patient had philosophical/religious reasons to refuse treatment, you might be on thin ice. Another alternative, and the mechanism tends to vary from state to state, is to petition a judge (generally in Superior Court) to grant a court order to treat the patient against his will. However, in these cases a lawyer will be appointed to represent the patient, and there may be some procedural delays. There are ways to overcome these delays, which hospital administrators know, but the process can be quite cumbersome and time consuming.

Most physicians would probably take measures to enforce at least lifesaving treatment in this case. There will be hurdles of course, the first being this patient's resistance, which will have to be countered with some form of restraint—physical, pharmacological, or both. In this particular case, there seems to be a good solution, which should also help with the other serious problem of incipient ethanol withdrawal: lorazepam intravenously for sedation. This can be given in doses of 2 mg and should be very effective for both issues. The next step is probably to start broad meningitis/encephalitis antimicrobial treatment and to quickly arrange for a CT scan of the head, followed (if there is no mass or hemorrhage intracranially) by LP.

KEY POINTS TO REMEMBER

- Patients have the right to refuse treatment.
- When you suspect that a patient has cognitive incapacity or a psychiatric condition that prevents understanding and/ or appreciation of the seriousness of the medical status, and consequences of refusing treatment, a determination of decision-making capacity should be made.
- A court order can be obtained to test or treat, but in emergencies, an exception is generally assumed to be granted.

Further Reading

Bernat JL. *Ethical Issues in Neurology.* 3rd ed. Philadelphia: Lippincott, Williams & Wilkins; 2008:27-30 and 182-184.

Grisso T, Appelbaum PS, Hill-Fotouhi C. The MacCAT-T: A clinical tool to assess patients' capacities to make treatment decisions. *Psychiatr Serv.* 1997;48:1415-1419.

Moberg PJ, Kniele K. Evaluation of competency: ethical considerations for neuropsychologists. *Applied Neuropsychol.* 2006;13:101-114.

23 Functional Paraparesis

A 37-year-old woman is transferred from another hospital for neurosurgical evaluation of acute bilateral leg weakness. She was well yesterday, but this morning at work, in her job as a secretary, she began to become weak in her lower extremities. This progressed over the course of the day and by midday she was unable to walk. She shared this with her coworkers who insisted she seek medical attention. She has never experienced similar symptoms and does not relate any recent trauma or back/leg pain. She thinks it might be due to her very uncomfortable chair at work. On exam, vital signs are normal, lungs are clear, cardiac exam is normal, abdomen is non-tender, and auscultation is benign. There is no spinal or back tenderness, limbs seem normal without deformity, and skin appears normal. Neurological exam reveals normal mental status exam, intact cranial nerves, and preserved reflexes in all limbs, without Babinski reflexes. Abdominal reflexes are present bilaterally. Motor tone is normal in all regions. Upper extremity motor function is normal. She is unable to move her legs more than small excursions. Hoover sign is present bilaterally. Sensation is reduced in her legs up to the inguinal ligament, but there are multiple areas in different dermatomes bilaterally that are sensitive to pain. Rectal tone is normal. Reached by phone, the neurosurgical consultant recommended a full-spine MRI scan, which has just been done and appears normal.

What do you do now?

This appears to be a psychogenic somatoform condition, but, of course, neurological disease needs to be ruled out. Patients with psychogenic paraplegia generally lie in bed unmoving. If they are convinced to attempt to walk, they may lurch dramatically and nearly fall. Once back in bed, they will often display better strength on manual motor testing. This is one of the most important ways to detect non-neurological weakness—looking for inconsistency. One can surreptitiously do this when the patient does not realize anyone is observing; video monitoring can be of use as well. Sensation is generally non-neurologic in pattern—the entire leg up to the groin (as with this patient), or to a demarcation point that is not in keeping with nerve or muscle anatomy and physiology. Reflexes are generally normal. And often the patient is relatively calm about the whole thing, demonstrating "la belle indifférence." Hoover's sign (failure to press downward with the strong leg when attempting to lift up the weak leg) is often positive, but with bilateral leg weakness, one would not expect to learn much from it. Collapsing or "give-way" weakness is another marker that is reasonably reliable. In this case, however, the patient is so weak she might not be able to even move a muscle with enough force that could then give way. Lifting the weak limb to see whether it will drop slower than normally, implying some antagonist muscle activity, can suggest functional weakness. One can take it a step further and see whether the dropping the limb in a dangerous way (letting an arm drop to the face if not checked) might elicit some motor activity. This is more difficult in the legs (see Table 23.1 for a list of clues to diagnosing functional weakness).

The exam and imaging findings seem to pretty much exclude a neurological cause of paraplegia. Spinal stroke can be missed on MRI and so

TABLE 23.1 **Clues to Functional Weakness**

Hoover's sign
Inconsistency of findings
Weakness or sensory symptoms in a nonphysiologically typical territory
Absence of reflex abnormality
Absence of bowel, bladder, or sensory level in paraplegia
Give-way weakness or "collapsing" strength
Dramatic gait abnormalities without falling
Avoidance of injury with hand-drop over face

might a vascular malformation. A new active MS plaque in the spinal cord could cause a similar syndrome, although the rapidity and severity of the paraparesis would be strange. Any of these might be present in the thoracic region and cause paraparesis with mixed sensory findings. Reflexes might be normal or diminished initially, due to the mechanism of "spinal shock," so exam may be deceiving. (Abdominal reflexes should disappear however, if the lesion is above T9). Somatosensory evoked potentials could help—if abnormal, a search for spinal pathology can continue, perhaps with spinal angiography. But again, with preserved abdominal and rectal reflexes, no incontinence, and the nonphysiological exam in general, this is almost certainly a functional condition.

Differentiating consciously produced and unconsciously produced functional symptoms is a bit more difficult. This is probably because a continuum exists here with some patients clearly aware and others only minimally aware that they are simulating signs and symptoms. If truly involuntary, as this patient's syndrome seems to be, the state is termed *Conversion Disorder*, which is one of the somatoform disorders described in the Diagnostic and Statistical Manual of Mental Disorders, Fourth edition, Text revision (DSM IV TR). With these patients, it is very important to make sure the diagnosis is shared in a nonjudgmental way. If it feels accusatory, it can be re-traumatizing to the patient, whose syndrome may be originating from significant trauma in the past. Instead, couching the explanation in terms of stress or anxiety may be very well-accepted. Most patients improve gradually, on their own, and it is a good idea to share this fact with patients such as the one presented here. Understanding family dynamics and even pursuing family counseling, as well as individual counseling, may be very helpful. Admission overnight is not reinforcing but rather lends a feeling of safety to the patient. Cognitive behavioral therapy is said to provide long-term benefits.

If this patient is consciously generating symptoms and signs, it will be important to determine the motive. If there is no particular reward for the patient other than being in the "sick role," this is *Factitious Disorder* and is rather akin to self-harm. These patients generally have psychiatric problems and often, like patients with conversion disorder, have a history of abuse. Factitious disorder tends to respond to some of the same approaches that are effective in conversion disorder, but it has a better prognosis. If the presentation seems clearly related to financial or other gain, it is *malingering* and not really a medical disorder at all. Malingering patients can be extremely difficult to manage, but there is no reason to hospitalize them because there is no risk of self-harm.

KEY POINTS TO REMEMBER

- Signs of functional weakness include Hoover's sign, give-way weakness, inconsistency of findings, and normal reflexes, but these can all be misleading on occasion.
- Patients with weakness on the basis of conversion disorder are entirely unconscious that there is no organic basis to their paresis.
- Patients with conscious gain in mind are malingering, and those who are producing symptoms in order to fit into a sick role have factitious disorder.

Further Reading

American Psychiatric Association. *Diagnostic and Statistical Manual of Mental Disorders, Fourth Edition, Text revision (DSM IV TR).* Washington DC: American Psychiatric Press, Inc; 2000.

McDermott BE, Feldman MD. Malingering in the medical setting. *Psychiatr Clin North Am.* 2007;30(4):645-662.

Williamson RT. The differential diagnosis between functional and organic paraplegia. *Br Med J.* 1918;2:275-277.

Zull DN, Cydulka R. Acute paraplegia: A presenting manifestation of aortic dissection. *Am J Med.* 1988;84:765-770.

24 Nonepileptic Spells

A 28-year-old former heroin addict is brought to the ED
after a series of "seizures" manifested by bilateral lower
extremity shaking movements and verbal outbursts.
A friend with her states this has happened in the past
"when doctors changed her medicine," and suspects this
has happened again. The patient is in a buprenorphine-
naloxone program and is also on several psychoactive
drugs including duloxetine, sertraline, and quetiapine.
While you are examining her, she has another spell
with head turning from side-to-side, cursing, singing a
recognizable song, and bilateral rhythmic leg-shaking.
There is no incontinence, and after about 3 minutes
the patient stops shaking, looks at you and asks "Did
I do it again?—You've got to give me something to
stop these seizures!" She is able to converse but is
agitated and repeatedly asks for something to "just
calm me down!" Vital signs are normal. She is wearing
a brace for a "sprained ankle" and has several areas
of ecchymosis, which she states are due to falls as a
result of her medication making her clumsy. She moves
all extremities well but is a bit dysarthric. General and
neurological exams are otherwise normal.

What do you do now?

This patient's ictal behavior is decidedly inconsistent with epileptic seizures—maintenance of consciousness despite bilateral clonic limb movements, immediate return to fully interactive communication purporting lack of memory of the event, singing, etc. However, before diagnosing nonepileptic spells, certain key steps must be taken. One suspects that previous medical records will be revealing of pertinent history. Metabolic screening as well as drug screening should be done, and if there are any neurological signs, CT of the head should rule out significant intracranial pathology. Here the dysarthria may qualify, so CT is probably indicated. Unfortunately, EEG will probably not be particularly helpful unless another spell happens during recording. This patient apparently carries the diagnosis of epilepsy; so, at least for now, the term pseudoseizures should be avoided to prevent what can turn into highly unpleasant confrontations.

Seizures such as the ones this patient has are best termed psychogenic nonepileptic seizures (PNES) to distinguish them from "organic" nonepileptic seizures. The latter term refer to conditions such as migraine, movement disorders, syncope, and TIAs, which can mimic epilepsy. PNES are more common than was once thought, although prevalence is difficult to measure. The condition arises from (1) a somatoform disorder, in which case it can be thought of as a form of "conversion"; (2) factitious disorder (motivated by the need to be "sick"); or (3) malingering. As with other conversion disorder symptoms, the nature of the psychiatric etiology is unclear. PNES are often seen in people who have suffered abuse or trauma. They are usually misdiagnosed as epilepsy and because it is hard to reverse that diagnosis, correct identification often takes years.

Often, PNES episodes manifest with behavior unusual in epileptic seizures, such as asynchronous limb-shaking, laughing, crying, arching of the back, and awareness of surroundings despite apparent bilateral cerebral discharges. Self-injury, such as tongue biting, which is common in epileptic generalized motor seizures, is less common, as is incontinence. Triggers for PNES spells tend to be emotional or situational, and usually occur in the presence of others. There is often a history of refractoriness to anticonvulsant medications, necessitating frequent medication changes. There is also commonly a history of post-traumatic stress disorder (PTSD) and childhood sexual and physical abuse.

Diagnosis of PNES rests on video-EEG monitoring, which is nearly always successful (if a spell is observed) in differentiating it from frontal-lobe epilepsy and from complex partial seizures that may resemble the behavioral manifestations of PNES. If this service is unavailable at your institution, it is relatively easy to find a referral epilepsy center. Once the diagnosis of PNES is made, the process of communicating this to the patient and designing a treatment program begins. This should be done in a nonjudgmental fashion, and be framed in such a way that it does not suggest that the patient is malingering, because that is usually not the case. Cognitive behavioral therapy is reported to be helpful. SSRI antidepressants have also been shown to be helpful in some patients.

When PNES patients who have already been diagnosed are seen in the ED following a spell or series of spells, the approach can still be problematic. There are often mixed feelings about the diagnosis, and more often than not, antiepileptic medication has been continued "just in case." This does nothing, of course, but confuse the patient and family. It then falls to the medical team in the ED to try to make some progress towards appropriate treatment. Again, approaching the diagnosis in a nonaccusatory way is essential in order to make any progress. Psychiatric consultation should be sought, and collection of previous video-EEG data can be very useful as well. It is important to avoid repetition of diagnostic testing and escalation of antiepileptic medication.

One issue that often surfaces on these occasions is the relatively inaccurate concept that many patients with PNES also have epileptic seizures, and that therefore both conditions should be assessed and treated aggressively. In fact, only a small percentage of PNES patients have epileptic seizures, estimated in epilepsy centers to be, at most, 10%. Here again, video-EEG monitoring is helpful but must sometimes be carried out over a longer time frame.

KEY POINTS TO REMEMBER

- The diagnosis of psychogenic nonepileptic seizures (PNES) is challenging and patients may be misdiagnosed with epilepsy for years.
- Clues to the diagnosis of PNES can be found in the ictal presentation, as well as in the patient's description of triggers.
- Video-EEG monitoring is generally successful in distinguishing PNES from epilepsy.
- Communicating the diagnosis to the patient must be done in a clear and consistent but nonaccusatory way.

Further Reading

Avbersek A, Sisodiya S. Does the primary literature provide support for clinical signs used to distinguish psychogenic nonepileptic seizures from epileptic seizures? *J Neurol Neurosurg Psychiatry.* 2010;81:719-725.

Carton S, Thompson PJ, Duncan JS. Non-epileptic seizures: patients' understanding and reaction to the diagnosis and impact on outcome. *Seizure.* 2003;12(5):287-294.

Goldstein LH, Chalder T, Chigwedere C, Khondoker MR, Moriarty J, Toone BK, et al. Cognitive-behavioral therapy for psychogenic nonepileptic seizures: a pilot RCT. *Neurology.* 2010;74(24):1986-1994.

Reuber M, Fernandez G, Bauer J, et al. Diagnostic delay in psychogenic nonepileptic seizures. *Neurology.* 2002;58(3):493-495.

25 Intracranial Mass Lesion in HIV Infection

A 40-year-old man with increasing confusion is seen in the ED and found on CT of the head to have a 3x4x4 cm right frontal lesion that enhances. He tested positive for HIV one month ago and has not been started on treatment. He has no primary care provider (PCP). He is an unemployed graphic designer. He smokes about one pack of cigarettes daily. He has no other complaints or known medical illnesses other than insomnia and excessive past alcohol use (recently rare according to the patient). General exam is normal except for some mild neck stiffness in all directions, and mildly elevated BP at 150/92. Mental status exam is normal except for some memory deficits (does poorly with naming within a category), decreased orientation skills (knows date but not day of the week or correct name of the hospital) and some difficulty with attentional tasks (e.g., digit span). Neurological exam is otherwise generally unremarkable except for a subtle pronator drift in the left arm. Reflexes are symmetrical. Gait is good and Romberg is negative.

What do you do now?

The differential diagnosis of a single mass is not terribly large, but it differs for patients with normal immune function as opposed to those with a compromised immune system, as in this patient. Location, and/or exposure to foreign locations, also plays a role. In patients with a normal immune system, the list includes glioma, metastatic tumors, multiple sclerosis plaque, bacterial abscess, cysticercosis (if there is a history of living in or travel to an endemic area), and sarcoidosis. In patients with AIDS, on chemotherapy, transplant patients, or patients immunosuppressed from other causes, the list should also include fungal abscess (e.g., Cryptococcus), lymphoma, tuberculosis, toxoplasmosis, and nocardia (see Table 25.1). Progressive multifocal leukoencephalopathy (PML) may also take the form of an apparent mass lesion in these patients. Clinical presentation does not help narrow the list very much, as most can present with headache, focal findings, and either seizures or depression of consciousness.

Imaging characteristics can be helpful. CT and MRI scanning with contrast can shed some light regarding different etiologies of mass lesions in these patients. Cerebral toxoplasmosis tends to produce contrast-enhancing single or multiple nodules with irregular margins and necrosis in the center,

TABLE 25.1 **Differential Diagnosis of Mass Lesion in Immunocompromised Patients**

Fungal abscess (Cryptococcus, Candida, Aspergillosis, Mucormycosis, Coccidiomycosis)

Bacterial abscess (Listeria, Treponema, Nocardia, Mycobacterium tuberculosis, Mycobacterium avium intracellulare)

Toxoplasmosis

Cysticercosis

Progressive multifocal leukoencephalopathy (PML)

CNS lymphoma

Kaposi sarcoma

Metastatic lesion

Glioma

Stroke

Intracerebral hemorrhage

Tumefactive multiple sclerosis

Sarcoidosis

with surrounding edema. Cerebral tuberculosis produces variably enhancing small nodules, without edema. On the other hand, larger tuberculosis abscesses can occur and resemble other bacterial abscesses. Brain abscesses are thick-walled with wall enhancement and significant edema. Lymphoma also shows enhancement with some edema.

These characteristics are not specific enough, however, to help the emergency room physician or neurologist map out a rational course for diagnosis and treatment. What are the best steps here? Large lesions with mass effect threatening herniation should signal the need for open biopsy with decompression. If this is not the case, it will be important to try to exclude some of the possibilities.

Positron emission tomography (PET) and SPECT can help to distinguish CNS lymphoma from infectious processes—lymphoma tends to reveal hypermetabolic features whereas infections are relatively hypometabolic. Chest radiography should help to exclude tuberculosis, and, especially in smokers, it may reveal lung neoplasms. Toxoplasma serology is generally positive in CNS toxoplasmosis. If it is positive, most would suggest empiric antibiotic treatment. The findings of lymphopenia (< 800 cell/mm) and low CD4+ counts generally suggest the presence of an opportunistic infection or malignancy (e.g., toxoplasmosis, cryptococcosis, PML, and lymphoma) while higher CD4+ counts make nonopportunistic microorganisms (e.g., tuberculosis, bacteria, Nocardia, and herpes simplex) more likely. CSF cytology can sometimes identify abnormal cells. The risks of lumbar puncture in a patient with intracranial masses are significant, however, and CSF samples in many of the infectious processes may yield only nonspecific pleocytosis and increased CSF protein. Bacterial abscesses tend to lead to more headache and malaise but can be indolent. Blood cultures and a search for an infectious source in the sinuses, ears, mouth and teeth, and heart should be done.

Taking this all into consideration, the best approach to the non-life-threatening intracranial mass lesion in HIV/AIDS is probably to check toxoplasmosis serology and attempt to obtain SPECT images. If toxoplasmosis serology is positive, treat empirically, particularly if SPECT shows a "cold" spot. If toxoplasmosis serology is negative, particularly if SPECT is suggestive of lymphoma, one could try corticosteroid treatment, which leads to shrinkage of primary CNS lymphomas in many cases. (Recurrence of primary CNS lymphoma always occurs unless chemotherapy and radiation therapy is added, but this initial treatment can be helpful in diagnosis and serve to improve symptoms quickly.) If either approach does not lead to improvement on imaging, or if there is high suspicion of bacterial abscess, stereotactic biopsy would be appropriate. No algorithm is perfect so clinical judgment and discussion with patients is crucial. And finally, of course, this patient needs to be treated for his HIV infection with antiretrovirals and have his leukocyte counts and general health closely monitored.

KEY POINTS TO REMEMBER

- While toxoplasmosis is the common etiology underlying intracranial mass lesions, a number of other infectious, neoplastic, and other processes may present in this way.
- Functional neuroimaging testing can help to distinguish between some of these conditions.
- Lumbar puncture in HIV-infected patients with intracranial mass lesions is generally unrevealing and can be risky.

Further Reading

American Academy of Neurology Quality Standards Committee. Evaluation and management of intracranial mass lesions in AIDS. *Neurology.* 1998:50:21-26.

Antinori A, Ammassari A, Luzzati R, et al. Role of brain biopsy in the management of focal brain lesions in HIV-infected patients. Gruppo Italiano Cooperativo AIDS & Tumori. *Neurology.* 2000;54:993.

Ruiz A, Ganz WI, Post MJ, et al. Use of thallium-201 brain SPECT to differentiate cerebral lymphoma from toxoplasma encephalitis in AIDS patients. *Am J Neuroradiol.* 1994;15:1885.

Stenzel W, Pels H, Staib P, et al. Concomitant manifestation of primary CNS lymphoma and Toxoplasma encephalitis in a patient with AIDS. *J Neurol.* 2004;251:764.

First Seizure

A 42-year-old man was seen earlier today to "look off into space," and "within a few minutes" was observed to have a generalized tonic-clonic seizure. He had urinary incontinence. He has had no recent illnesses or medical symptoms. He has been working long hours lately and is sleep deprived. He has no history of seizures or stroke. CT of the head was normal as was a lumbar puncture. He is very anxious. Vital signs are normal except for tachycardia at 110. Blood count reveals a WBC of 12,000, but differential count, red blood cell count, hematocrit, and hemoglobin are normal, as are serum chemistries. Full neurological exam is entirely normal.

What do you do now?

The initial question in a patient with a first-time seizure is: "Is this an epileptic seizure?" It certainly sounds like it, but it is important to remember that a number of conditions can mimic seizures, including movement disorders, TIAs, syncope, psychiatric conditions, and migraine. None of these seems likely here.

When patients do not recover from their seizure completely, have a prolonged postictal period (i.e., more than a couple of hours), have multiple seizures, are sick medically, or have an unstable/unsupervised home life, hospitalization is probably warranted. This patient, who apparently has none of these complicating issues, probably will be anxious to return home, which is not unreasonable. But the neurologist, who may never see this patient again, has a responsibility to attempt to predict the future and do everything possible to rule out treatable causes of seizures and to prevent seizure recurrence.

The white blood count elevation is entirely expected, as generalized seizures lead to WBC demargination and spuriously increased WBC counts, but infections should be considered. Other etiological factors should be entertained, such as intracranial mass lesions, meningitis, encephalitis, electrolyte imbalance, medication side effects (e.g., opioids, antidepressants), intoxication (particularly with stimulants) or withdrawal (see Table 26.1). Here, again, none of these seems likely. Sleep deprivation is likely to have contributed, but it is not the etiology. Autoimmune diseases of the brain, genetic diseases, perinatal cortical injury, and the remote effects of brain trauma are possibilities. To be certain no causative factors have been missed, the patient should have an MRI of the brain with and without contrast, and an EEG with provocative maneuvers such as photic stimulation and hyperventilation. Both of these procedures can generally safely be done during the subsequent several days on an outpatient basis, and hospital admission is not needed to expedite workup. After normal CT imaging of the brain, lumbar puncture is warranted in patients with fever, meningismus, or focality on neurological exam, including persistent alteration in mental status.

The decision about starting anticonvulsant medication in a patient who had a first seizure revolves around the risk of seizure recurrence, which is probably just below 50% on average, but changes depending on risk factors. One risk factor for seizure recurrence is partial onset—and here there

TABLE 26.1 **Causes of First-time Seizures**

- Intracranial neoplasm
- Brain abscess
- Subdural hematoma
- Cerebral infarction
- Intracerebral hemorrhage
- Cerebral venous thrombosis
- Meningitis
- Encephalitis
- Electrolyte imbalance (such as hyponatremia, hypocalcemia, hypoglycemia, uremia)
- Medication side effects (opioids, antidepressants)
- Drug intoxication (amphetamines, cocaine)
- Drug withdrawal (barbiturates, benzodiazepines)
- Ethanol withdrawal
- Cerebral vasculitis
- Perinatal cortical injury
- Post-traumatic cortical injury
- Inherited metabolic diseases

seems to have been partial complex activity followed by secondary generalization. Other risk factors are the presence of focal neurological deficits on exam, the presence of epileptiform activity on EEG, and brain CT or MRI abnormalities. With normal MRI, the risk of a recurrence after the first seizure goes down to about 30%. Other considerations, of course, are the relative risks and benefits of anticonvulsant medication for the particular patient. Some neurologists ask patients about their lifestyle risks—that is, the consequences of a seizure recurrence. For example, a seizure recurrence in a long-distance truck driver might be of more concern than in an office worker. However, ANY generalized seizure is potentially life-threatening, particularly if it should happen while the patient is driving, on a stairway, etc. The decision is, therefore, individualized and should be made as a team with input from the patient, family, and neurologist. Often, if workup is entirely normal, instituting anticonvulsant therapy is done with the plan of tapering and stopping medication within a year if seizures have not recurred and EEG remains normal. This might be reasonable here. Equally reasonable, if the patient wishes, the decision can be postponed until the EEG and further brain imaging has been done. And it is not unreasonable to simply choose to adjust lifestyle to raise the seizure "threshold" and avoid taking anticonvulsants entirely for the time being. For the patient presented above, this would involve ensuring adequate sleep, avoiding intoxicants such as ethanol, and probably looking into stress-reducing tactics, including personal counseling. Most neurologists would agree that anticonvulsant treatment is indicated after two seizures, as recurrence risk is significantly higher after two or more unprovoked seizures than after just one, rising to 70% even in patients with normal brain MRI scans.

The best choice in anticonvulsant medication for a first-time generalized seizure is not clear. Several studies have attempted to compare the available anticonvulsants on the basis of effectiveness and tolerance, but different results seem to surface. All antiepileptic drugs can potentially have fairly significant side effects, and many alter hepatic metabolic activity. Some should be titrated upward slowly, which will lead to a delay in attaining therapeutic levels. Serum drug concentrations can be useful with some anticonvulsants but not all. One can think of most of the current AEDs in two broad categories:

1. Those effective against partial seizures (focal seizures) as well as generalized seizures that begin focally—including carbamazepine, phenytoin, phenobarbital, gabapentin, and oxcarbamazepine
2. Those effective against both initially generalized and partial seizures—including valproate, lamotrigine, topiramate, levetiracetam, and zonisamide

Given that little is yet known about this patient's seizure type, other than it became generalized, a good choice might be to begin levetiracetam (Keppra®) at a dose of 250 mg bid with increase in 2 weeks to 500 mg bid. The dose can be much higher if clinical judgment warrants. Other good choices are valproate and topiramate. It is essential to know and share with patients the common adverse effects of AEDs you are considering and to alert them to whatever monitoring lab tests will be necessary.

It is worth letting patients know that around 10% of people will have one seizure, and about 1% have epilepsy (recurrent unprovoked seizures). And that after having had one seizure, however, there is a higher risk of having a second seizure. Based on this, many patients will opt to start an

AED, at least for several months. Whatever is decided, the patient should be cautioned about risks of driving, operating machinery, or performing any activity that might be dangerous to himself or others if he were to have a seizure. You should be aware of state laws concerning cessation of driving after documented seizure occurrence and counsel the patient about his/her responsibilities concerning this, as well as any requirement to notify stated motor vehicle departments.

KEY POINTS TO REMEMBER

- First-time seizures should trigger an extensive workup to exclude intracranial pathology and metabolic causes.
- The acute evaluation of a patient with a first-time seizure should include CT scan of the brain, and preferably, EEG, as well as full metabolic evaluation including toxicology.
- MRI of the brain, and possibly LP, should also be done in the near future.
- The decision to begin seizure prophylaxis after a first seizure depends on the patient's risks, preferences, and results of the workup, particularly MRI and EEG.

Further Reading

Berg AT, Berkovic SF, Brodie MJ, et al. Revised terminology and concepts for organization of seizures and epilepsies: report of the ILAE Commission on Classification and Terminology, 2005-2009. *Epilepsia*. 2010;51:676-685.

Bonnet LJ, Shukralla A, Tudur-Smith C, Williamson PR, Marson AG. Seizure recurrence after antiepileptic drug withdrawal and the implications for driving: further results from the MRC Antiepileptic Drug Withdrawal Study and a systematic review. *J Neurol Neurosurg Psychiatry*. 2011;82:1328-1333.

Chadwick DW. The treatment of the first seizure: the benefits. *Epilepsia*. 2008;49(suppl 1): 26-28.

Hesdorffer DC, Benn EKT, Cascino GD, Hauser WA. Is a first acute symptomatic seizure epilepsy? Mortality and risk for recurrent seizure. *Epilepsia*. 2009;50:1102-1108.

PART IV

Pediatric Dilemmas in Neurology

Severe Headache in a Child with Migraine

A 25-kg 9-year-old boy with recurrent migraine headaches awoke with a particularly severe headache this morning. He has been vomiting all morning and has been unresponsive to oral analgesics and antiemetics. IM ketoralac has been only minimally helpful. IM prochlorperazine has helped the nausea, but severe headache persists. General and neurological exams are normal. CT has not been done to avoid exposure to radiation.

What do you do now?

This boy seems to have a typical case of migraine, which is not uncommon. (Before puberty, male and female prevalence of migraine is roughly equal). But the extreme severity is unusual. The unremitting vomiting and intractability of the pain is also a bit unusual but not unheard of. Thorough neurological examination, including comprehensive mental status exam, should be performed to make sure there really is no focal deficit. If this is normal, then a CT scan is probably not necessary. An MRI is probably worthwhile at some point to exclude intracranial mass, arteriovenous malformation, and congenital cranial malformations such as Arnold Chiari. The general examination should focus on evidence of trauma, accidental or inflicted, as well as any signs of infection or general medical issues. He should be screened carefully for meningismus. It is important to check basic metabolic function regarding electrolyte balance (especially given the persistent vomiting), glucose level, blood counts, and hepatic and renal function. Ruling out infection is crucial because urinary, pulmonary, ear, and other infections can induce severe migraine.

A good first step in treating this boy is to make sure to replace lost fluids IV. This will provide the added benefit of IV access for potentially useful pain and nausea-relieving medications. Other than the neuroleptic/anti-emetics, medications that might be useful for the nausea include ondansetron and hydroxyzine. Ondansetron is available as a sublingual 4 mg or 8 mg wafer that children often tolerate well, although it is not known to be entirely safe in this patient's age group. The dose is in the .15 mg/kg range. Hydroxyzine is an antihistaminic that has both antiemetic and analgesic, as well as anxiolytic, properties, and can be given intramuscularly as well as intravenously in a dosage of approximately .25–.5 mg/kg.

Other than for acetaminophen and ibuprofen, there is very little evidence of safety or efficacy of any acute antimigraine medication in children. While ergots are not known to be safe in children, DHE in a dose of approximately .25 mg IV for preteens, and .5–1.0 mg for teens, has been used successfully. A less potent approach, which might be better tolerated, is the nasal form marketed as Migranal®. In this age group, it could probably be taken as one spray in each nostril. An antinauseant should be used along with DHE because it can be nauseating. Almotriptan has been approved for use in adolescents, and although not officially approved, several other triptans have been shown in controlled blinded studies to be effective in adolescents—sumatriptan in the nasal form at a dose of 20 mg, zolmitriptan nasal 5 mg, and rizatriptan and almotriptan in the oral forms at 5 and 6.25 mg respectively. Subcutaneous sumatriptan has been used successfully in adolescents and children, but it is hard to adjust dosage appropriately because it comes in a prefilled canister.

Finally, most children and adolescents will find that the migraine resolves after sleep. Most of the antinauseants have some soporific effects so they can be used. Good choices include promethazine 0.5–1 mg/kg orally or rectally, and prochlorperazine 0.15 mg/kg in parenteral, rectal, or oral forms. It is important to remember that dyskinesia can occur. Hydroxyzine likewise has a sedative effect; an alternative is dimenhydramine (Benadryl®) in a dose of .5–1 mg/kg in oral or parenteral forms. In rare cases, none of these seem to work and deeper sedation may be needed, which can be achieved with barbiturates or opioids. If this approach is necessary, it should probably be done on an inpatient basis so that the patient can be observed carefully.

Most children with severe migraine are to some extent scared or nervous about the intensity of the acute experiences. Counseling can help, and this also opens the door for family counseling, which could help to reduce triggers and defuse some of the drama for all family members that can escalate during the acute attacks. Screening for medication overuse is essential. If headaches are frequent, lead to frequent ED visits, or lead to missed social or family events, the use of preventive measures must be considered, and a referral to a pediatric neurologist/headache specialist probably is warranted.

KEY POINTS TO REMEMBER

- With severe migraine in a child, secondary causes must be ruled out, including neurological infections, intracranial mass, and systemic metabolic or infectious disease.
- There is little evidence to aid in choosing agents for acute migraine treatment in children.
- Triptans can be very effective for childhood migraine, as can antinauseants and sedatives.
- Most children with severe recurrent migraine headaches find them to be emotionally stressful and can benefit from counseling and family counseling.

Further Reading

Hershey AD, Winner P. Pediatric migraine: recognition and treatment. *J Am Osteopath Assoc.* 2005;105:2S-8S.

Lewis D, Ashwal S, Hershey A, Hirtz D, Yonker M, Silberstein S. Pharamacological treatment of migraine headache in children and adolescents. Report of the American Academy of Neurology Quality Standards Subcommittee and the Practice Committee of the Child Neurology Society. *Neurology.* 2004;63:2215-2224.

Richer LP, Laycock K, Millar K, et al. Treatment of children with migraine in emergency departments: national practice variation study. *Pediatrics.* 2010;126:e150-e155.

28 Febrile Seizure

A 4-year-old girl is brought to the ED after having a generalized seizure in her sleep. Her mother, who is a nurse, witnessed the seizure and describes diffuse body stiffening, followed by generalized limb-shaking. The mother relates that her daughter seemed to stop breathing and looked "cyanotic." The seizure lasted approximately 15 minutes and was followed by mild somnolence, which has persisted now for 1 hour. She recently had a gastrointestinal viral syndrome with diarrhea and vomiting, accompanied by fever up to 103° F, but she has only had "at most" a mild fever over the past 12 hours, according to the mother.

What do you do now?

B enign febrile seizures generally occur in children between 3 months and 5 years of age. The incidence is probably between 5% and 10%. These seizures are usually single, generalized, and last less than 15 minutes. The child should be otherwise neurologically healthy and without neurological abnormality by examination or by developmental history. If there is any focality to the seizure, if it is prolonged, or if there are any focal neurological findings on exam, it does not qualify as a "simple febrile seizure" (see Table 28.1.)

In this case, a couple of features are a bit unsettling. First, the seizure was rather prolonged. Fifteen minutes is still within the "simple" febrile seizure window, but it is at the upper limit. The mother should be a good historian because she is a nurse, but parents may overestimate the duration of seizures; the actual duration may have been shorter. It is not clear whether this child was febrile at the time. But most important, she is not returning to completely normal consciousness. This could be explained, however, by the time of night—occurring in the middle of her normal sleep cycle. The cyanosis is actually not that uncommon, with some children seemingly becoming apneic for a short time.

The most important question to ask is whether this seizure could be due to meningitis or encephalitis. LP, while not usually necessary for simple febrile seizures, would not be a bad idea here. There is scant risk of causing brain herniation with a nonfocal neurological exam, but CT of the head could easily be done to rule out a mass. Since serum glucose will be drawn to compare with CSF glucose, checking electrolytes, calcium, and perhaps magnesium, along with a CBC is probably worth doing as well, even though this is generally not necessary in patients with benign febrile seizures. LP is particularly worthwhile in infants between 6 and 12

TABLE 28.1 **Features of "Simple" Febrile Seizures**

- Febrile at the time of the seizure
- Single seizure
- Age between 3 months and 5 years
- Generalized without evidence of focality
- Duration less than 15 minutes
- Normal neurological exam
- Normal developmental history

months of age who have not received the usual Haemophilus influenzae or Streptococcus pneumoniae immunizations and who present with a seizure and fever.

Once CNS infection is ruled out, it might be worthwhile to search further for a structural cause for the seizure. However, in cases where febrile seizures do not recur, and the patient fully awakens with no residual deficits, MRI scanning of the brain is not considered necessary. An EEG might provide some evidence of an epileptic focus in rare patients with febrile seizures, but it is probably not indicated in this patient either. If she awakens fully, if CSF is normal, and no abnormalities are seen on the basic blood testing, there is also no reason to admit her to the hospital.

Finally, questions regarding future seizure risk and the need for prophylactic treatment generally arise. Patients with simple febrile seizures have only a slightly higher risk of recurrent seizures (unless they recur during a fever in the right age range) than any other person. Children with "complex febrile seizures" (i.e., those not fulfilling the requirements for simple febrile seizures) are much more likely, probably in the range of 80%, to have epilepsy later. Given that this patient essentially falls within the benign febrile seizure group, she should not have a significantly increased risk of seizure recurrence. Prophylaxis with antiepileptic medication is generally not recommended for children who have had a single febrile seizure; the benefit is low and there are significant side effects to all antiepileptic medications. If the parents' concern is high, EEG can be helpful in identifying any potential seizure focus that might suggest prophylactic treatment.

KEY POINTS TO REMEMBER

- Simple febrile seizures generally do not require lab investigation.
- If there is any suggestion of meningitis or encephalitis, lumbar puncture should be strongly considered.
- Focal seizure activity, prolonged duration of the seizure (> 15 minutes), multiple seizures, older age (> 5 years), or abnormal neurological exam should prompt a more careful investigation.
- Prophylaxis is not indicated for single simple febrile seizures.

Further Reading

American Academy of Pediatrics Subcommittee on Febrile Seizures. Neurodiagnostic evaluation of the child with a simple febrile seizure: clinical practice guideline. *Pediatrics.* 2011;127:389-394.

Dubea C, Brewster AL, Baram TZ. Febrile seizures: mechanisms and relationship to epilepsy. *Brain Dev.* 2009;31:366-371.

Shinnar S, Glauser TA. Febrile seizures. *J Child Neurol.* 2002;17(suppl 1):s44-s52.

Sillanpää M, Camfield P, Camfield C. Incidence of febrile seizures in Finland: prospective population-based study. *Pediatr Neurol.* 2008;38:391-394.

29 Acute Ataxia in a Child

A 6-year-old girl is brought to the ED by her mother because of gait difficulty. She had been well until yesterday when she began stumbling while walking, and when she tried to play with her dog she kept falling. She has no other symptoms and general exam is normal with BP 90/60, pulse regular at 76, respirations 14, and temperature of 98° F. Birth and past medical history are unremarkable, and there is no family history of neurological disease. On neurological exam, mental status seems entirely intact and she is not upset. Cranial nerves are also normal except for some dysarthria, which the mother and child notice as well. Horizontal nystagmus on end gaze in both directions is also seen. Motor tone and strength are intact, as is sensation. Reflexes are all present and symmetrical. Gait is clearly dysfunctional with incoordination of limbs as well as truncal instability. CT of the head is entirely normal.

What do you do now?

Differential diagnosis of the acute cerebellar syndrome in children (Table 29.1) includes intracranial fossa mass lesions, such as cerebellar astrocytoma, neuroblastoma, medulloblastoma, or abscess, and posterior fossa subdural or intraparenchymal hemorrhages. A CT scan of the head should rule most of these out, but MRI with contrast is the most reliable imaging test if deemed necessary. A posterior fossa mass seems unlikely in this case, however, given the rather acute nature of this presentation. Meningitis and encephalitis must also be excluded so these patients should probably have CSF analyzed. Acute disseminated encephalomyelitis (ADEM) is a rare cause of ataxia without other symptoms, but it can occur. MRI in ADEM should be abnormal and CSF should have a high protein level, with possibly a few mononuclear leukocytes. Accidental ingestion of medication such as anticonvulsants can lead to ataxia, and some detective work along these lines might be fruitful. Toxins such as ethanol or illicit drugs can also lead to cerebellar dysfunction and must be excluded. Although this patient does not have the typical back pain and lower extremity weakness seen in spinal cord lesions such as discitis, myelopathy with sensory and/or motor dysfunction should be kept in mind as a cause of apparent ataxia.

The Miller Fisher syndrome, which is considered a variant of Guillain-Barré syndrome, may present with acute cerebellar symptoms and signs, but should be accompanied by hyporeflexia and ophthalmoplegia. The opsoclonus/myoclonus syndrome is another possibility, also known as "dancing eyes-dancing feet." This is a paraneoplastic autoimmune disorder seen in children with

TABLE 29.1 **Causes of Acute Childhood Ataxia**

Cerebellar tumor
Cerebellar abscess
Cerebellar hemorrhage
Posterior fossa subdural hematoma
Opsoclonus/myoclonus syndrome
Miller Fisher syndrome
Labyrinthitis
Medication effect
Toxins
Discitis or other cause of myelopathy
Postinfectious acute childhood ataxia

neuroblastoma. It manifests as migratory myoclonic jerks and dramatic jumping eye movements (opsoclonus) as well as ataxia. This patient did have mild nystagmus but did not have the prerequisite opsoclonic movements or myoclonic jerks. Acute labyrinthitis can lead to the appearance of ataxia, and children might not be able to explain that their balance/gait difficulties stem from vertigo rather than imbalance. Nausea is usually preeminent, however, and children are generally quite distressed, as are adults, with vertigo.

Psychogenic gait disturbance (conversion disorder) is distinctly unusual in young children but should be kept in mind as a possibility. Risk factors include family stress and abuse, but it usually occurs in older children between 10 and 15 years of age.

When other more ominous possibilities are ruled out, the postinfectious benign syndrome of *acute cerebellar ataxia* is likely. This has been observed following a number of infections including varicella, Epstein-Barr virus, mycoplasma, enterovirus, roseola, rubeola, and parvovirus. The syndrome is generally seen in seen in children between 2 and 7 years old but has been reported in a few older children and adults. It probably accounts for about 40%–50% of the cases of acute ataxia in children. The mechanism is presumably immune-mediated cerebellar inflammation, and there have also been cases of acute ataxia in children who have recently had vaccinations. The child is generally unconcerned about the syndrome—much less so than parents. Other than truncal and limb ataxia with gait difficulty, there are generally no other accompanying symptoms. Some children have nystagmus as did this child. Symptoms begin to remit in several days in the majority of cases, so watching carefully is a reasonable approach once serious life-threatening causes are ruled out.

KEY POINTS TO REMEMBER

- Acute childhood ataxia is often due to a benign self-limited postinfectious condition.
- Accurate history is important to assure that the ataxia is acute rather than gradually progressive, and to rule out accidental ingestions and accompanying symptoms.
- Workup of acute ataxia in a child should include head CT or MRI, and possibly LP.

Further Reading

Salas AA, Nava A. Acute cerebellar ataxia in childhood: initial approach in the emergency department. *Emerg Med J.* 2010;27:956–957.

Van der Maas NAT, Vermeer-de Bondt PE, de Melker H, Kemmeren JM. Acute cerebellar ataxia in the Netherlands: a study on the association with vaccinations and varicella zoster infection. *Vaccine.* 2009;27:1970–1973.

30 Confusion in Childhood with Possible Abuse

An 8-year-old boy is brought to the ED by his father who states "he is not acting right." This began yesterday and has persisted, manifested by confused questions like "What is happening?" and "Is this a dream?" He could not go to school today and seemed to be stumbling. There have been no recent illnesses and his father states that he is "perfectly healthy." The ED staff noted some bruises of different ages on the boy's legs and a laceration on his right forearm. The father states that he does not know about these injuries, but that his son is very "active." He also has some neck pain with rotational movement. General exam is otherwise unremarkable. On neurological exam, mental status is reasonably good, but the patient tells you "nothing seems real." Orientation, memory, and language are all normal. Cranial nerves are intact, strength is good, sensation testing is grossly normal but seems confusing to him. Reflexes are normal and symmetrical, but you notice some pain with manipulation of the left arm. Gait is slightly clumsy but improves with repeated trials. CT of the head reveals a small contusion in the right frontal lobe without mass effect.

What do you do now?

This child's mental status is clearly altered. Possible causes include the frontal contusion, a psychiatric condition, a postictal state, a toxic or metabolic disturbance, or a CNS infection such as viral encephalitis. The neck pain on rotation is not typical for meningismus, and in the absence of a fever it is unlikely he has meningitis. So LP is probably not essential and, in fact, might be of some risk due to the small possibility of increased intracranial pressure, which could lead to shift of intracranial contents after LP. Ongoing partial seizure activity or postictal state are possibilities, but he seems to be fully alert despite feeling rather detached, which would be unusual in these states. MRI of the brain should be done to rule out other intracranial lesions, old or new. EEG would be of interest, but the yield is probably going to be low. Urine toxicology screen is mandatory and so is a full metabolic and hematologic profile (electrolytes, calcium, magnesium, glucose, BUN, creatinine, liver enzymes, CPK, CBC, PT and PTT).

If this workup is all negative, one can ascribe much of this child's behavior to the frontal contusion. There are, however, obvious clues pointing to abuse that must be sorted out in a careful but thorough fashion. The bruises, laceration, pain with movement of the left arm, and neck pain on movement should be documented and evaluated radiologically to rule out fracture. Physical abuse should be high on your list of possibilities but it is by no means certain. The lack of detail about recent injuries is, of course, suspicious in itself, and it is not unusual for children to be accompanied by the adult who has abused them.

Physical abuse is, of course, only one of the four types of abuse we need to be trained to detect. The other three are sexual abuse, psychological abuse, and neglect. In the case here, signs of physical abuse are abundant. A very thorough search, including a careful abdominal exam, should be undertaken, however, to detect hidden physical injuries. Sexual abuse may have occurred and emergency department personnel should be trained to document evidence of this, if there is any, via careful rectal and genital exams. Lab data can help determine whether there has been neglect of overall health. Psychological abuse is difficult to detect, but there is a strong suggestion of that here, as this child is displaying the state of derealization. Patients experiencing derealization frequently report highly unpleasant dreamlike or unreal feelings, as this child does, that do not resolve despite reassurance and distraction.

In summary, we need to be able to perform the following actions when confronted with suspected abuse:

1. Establish the diagnosis of probable abuse and of which type(s)
2. Document findings
3. Treat injuries
4. Address immediate safety issues
5. Report to appropriate child protective agency and/or law enforcement
6. Decide about inpatient versus outpatient care and eventual follow-up care

In this case, admission for neurological monitoring and psychiatric consultation seems essential. Careful lab and radiological testing to diagnose (and document) all medical and surgical problems must be done as soon as possible. Neurosurgical consultation must be done proactively in case expansion of the frontal contusion leads to a need to monitor pressure or perform surgery. Child protective services should be called immediately and the child should not be left alone at any time. Suspicions should not be voiced to the parent, but questions about any abuse will have to be asked eventually of him and anyone else available. This should be done in such a way as to avoid tainting the investigation.

KEY POINTS TO REMEMBER

- There are four types of abuse we need to be able to diagnose— physical, sexual, psychological, and neglect.
- Signs of physical abuse are easiest to detect and treat, and should prompt the investigation of other types of abuse.
- We have a responsibility to keep the possibly abused child safe.
- We have a responsibility to notify child protective services.

Further Reading

Jenny C, Hymel KP, Ritzen A, et al. Analysis of missed cases of abusive head trauma. *JAMA*. 1999;281(7):621-626.

Keshavarz R. Kawashima R. Low C. Child abuse and neglect presentations to a pediatric emergency department. *J Emerg Med*. 2002;23:341-345.

Louwers E, Korfage IJ, Affourtit M. Detection of child abuse in emergency departments: a multi-centre study. *Arch Dis Child*. 2011;96:422-425.

31 Concussion

A 16-year-old boy is brought to the ED by his soccer coach after an injury on the practice field 2 hours ago. His head collided with the shoulder of another player, when both attempted to head the ball, and the patient was knocked to the ground. He may have had a brief loss of consciousness, but was able to get up and slowly come off the field on his own. He was seen to "wander around" the sidelines for the next 30 minutes and was generally confused and disoriented after practice ended. He is still seen by the ED staff to be confused and you are called to evaluate him. General exam including vital signs is normal, although there seems to be some echymosis and tenderness in the left frontotemporal scalp. CT of the brain is negative. Mental status exam is remarkable for some disorientation to date and time, and poor memory for events during and after soccer practice. His speech seems a bit slow, but language is otherwise intact. Cranial nerves, motor tone and strength, sensation, coordination, and balance are all intact. The coach wants to know if it is "OK if he plays in the championship game tomorrow?"

What do you do now?

Concussion is defined as a change in neuropsychiatric function after a blow to the head. There need not be a loss of consciousness. Clearly there is a spectrum of severity to acute post-head-injury syndromes and many researchers have attempted to quantify symptoms and signs following injury in an effort to plan best treatment and predict recovery for each patient. But this has proven difficult. One conclusion seems clear—even mild head injuries can lead to lasting sequelae.

It is important to rule out epidural, subdural, and intracerebral hemorrhage in these patients as soon as possible. CT is very sensitive and, as in the case above, usually definitively rules these out. The tenderness over the frontotemporal scalp is unsettling because this is the general vicinity of the middle meningeal artery, which is the most common artery to cause epidural hematoma when lacerated. Interestingly, epidural hematomata actually may present with the classic pattern of loss of consciousness, a lucid interval, and then progressive deterioration, so this history is crucial to obtain. On the topic, skull fractures can be missed, but must be discovered because they can lead to very serious sequelae of CNS infection, later bleeding, and cranial nerve damage. Raccoon eyes (periorbital echymosis), Battle's sign (echymosis over the mastoid), otorrhea, and rhinorrhea are suggestive of basal skull fracture, but careful review of inferior views on the head CT is also imperative. Of course, careful assessment of the neurological exam with special attention to the cranial nerves is essential.

In patients with normal head CT scans, all is still not worry-free. Petechial hemorrhaging might have occurred, generally in anterior frontal or anterior temporal regions due to the net result of force vectors resulting from trauma, and this can progress. When these small areas of bleeding occur, they are often not apparent on initial CT scanning, and they can later coalesce and become true cerebral contusions, sometimes 24–48 hours later. These contusions can then lead to increased intracranial pressure and focal neurological deficits. Thus, repeating CT scans when patients seem to regress, or even if they do not clearly recover to their baseline, makes sense, as does screening blood count and bleeding parameters in patients who have sustained head injury.

So, assuming that all of the important workup is negative, can this young man return to play tomorrow? A consensus statement published by the *British Journal of Sports Medicine* suggests that any athlete, age 18 and under, who may have sustained a concussion during sports should not be allowed to return to activity the same day. In the past, this group believed that it was appropriate for the athlete to return to activity if cleared by a doctor or certified athletic trainer. The change came about when it became clear that there is no way to make an immediate determination of safety. The American Academy of Neurology (AAN) published a Practice Parameter in 1997 that attempted to codify how to make these decisions, and a 2010 position statement released by the AAN (www.aan.com) advised that (1) athletes who have had a concussion be removed from participation until evaluated by a physician who has had training in sports concussion; and (2) the concussed athlete not participate in sports if there are ANY persistent symptoms from the concussion and NOT return to participation until cleared by a physician with training in sports concussion. Numerous researchers have attempted to refine and direct treatment, return-to-play guidelines, and prognosis based upon symptoms and signs of patients following concussion, such as amnesia, headache, cognitive dysfunction, balance, etc. Unfortunately these all tend to occur and seem not be good predictors of future status. For example, virtually all concussed patients develop some retro- and anterograde amnesia, much of which resolves.

A number of patients will have persistent symptoms of the "postconcussive syndrome," which can last for months or even indefinitely, including headaches, dizziness, cognitive difficulties, sleep abnormalities, fatigue, and mood disturbances. These symptoms can either singly or as a whole become disabling, leading to falling behind in school and a great deal of emotional suffering. The cause(s) of these symptoms is not well understood but is being actively investigated, in large part due to the growing number of returning soldiers, concussed in combat as well as noncombat areas. One tool is diffusion tensor imaging (DTI), a MRI technique, which is being used to assess changes in white matter, thought by many to bear the brunt of force vectors delivered to the head. This and other imaging testing is also being correlated with neuropsychiatric testing pre- and post-athletic-season in an attempt to quantify cognitive changes. Of course, the athletes who are being tested are often canny enough to know that if they show a significant drop in cognition over the season, their coach may be reluctant to play them next year. As a result, preseason test scores can be artificially low.

At any rate, this patient certainly cannot go back to the field today. He may even need to be admitted to the hospital for careful observation and if he does not improve, perhaps a repeat CT scan of the head is called for to ensure that contusions have not formed. If he is entirely back to normal tomorrow, the question about return to play will be a difficult one. One important thing to always consider is that, for reasons still unclear, a second head injury can be devastating. To be safe, most would consider this patient to be best served by some time away from contact sports. How long is not clear.

KEY POINTS TO REMEMBER

- Concussion is defined as a change in neuropsychiatric function after a blow to the head, with or without loss of consciousness.
- Severe sequelae of head injury, such as epidural, subdural, and intracerebral hematomata must be ruled out acutely.
- Cerebral contusions can be delayed and should be investigated if the patient does not improve or regresses.
- There is recent consensus that returning to the field the same day after a sports injury is contraindicated.

Further Reading

Cantu RC. Guidelines for return to contact sports after a cerebral concussion. *Physician Sports Med.* 1986;14:75-83.

Kelly JP, Rosenberg JH. The diagnosis and management of concussion in sports. *Neurology.* 1997;48:575-580.

McCerory P, Meeuwisse W, Johnston K, et al. Consensus Statement on Concussion in Sport: the 3rd International Conference on Concussion in Sport. *Br J Sports Med.* 2009;43(suppl I):i76-i84.

Quality Standards Subcommittee of the American Academy of Neurology. Practice parameter: the management of concussion in sports. www.aan.com. 1997.

32 Acute Stroke in an Adolescent

A 15-year-old African-American girl acutely developed left-sided arm and leg weakness and is now being seen in the ED about 90 minutes after the onset of symptoms. CT of the head is normal. Routine labs are also normal according to the ED staff. Left-sided mild lower facial droop is seen, and there is mild dysarthria. Visual fields are fine, and body sensation is good as well. Left-sided 4/5 motor weakness is seen in the following muscles: ileopsoas, hamstring, quadriceps, anterior tibialis, and extensor hallucis longus. There was subtle weakness in the left upper extremity with pronator drift. Sensation seemed normal, but she said the "whole left side feels strange." Reflexes were roughly symmetrical. Gait was impaired due to the left leg weakness.

What do you do now?

S troke can occur in children and adolescents for the same major reasons that adults succumb: atherothrombosis and embolism. Although the risks are much lower, stroke in adolescence is not rare. A major cause of stroke in children and adolescents, much less common in adults, is sickle cell disease. This results from spontaneous thrombosis that can occur in any cerebral vessel. Sickle C disease is rarely a risk, and sickle trait does not lead to an increased risk of stroke. Leukemia can also lead to stroke. Neuroblastoma and other childhood neoplasms can also cause hypercoagulability, which can predispose to arterial or venous thrombosis. Inflammatory bowel disease also predisposes to stroke on probably the same basis. Cerebral venous thrombosis can also arise due to dehydration, infections of the ears, nose, sinuses, and meninges, and oral estrogen-containing medications. Vasculitis can occur in the setting of pharyngitis, sinusitis, chickenpox, pneumonia, syphilis, or tuberculosis, as well as with drug abuse.

Moya Moya and Takayasu diseases involve congenital arterial occlusions and lead to thrombotic strokes. Cyanotic heart disease will lead to child-hood stroke in many patients. Trauma to the carotid or vertebral arteries can cause arterial dissection and stroke. As in adulthood, lupus, and other collagen vascular disorders such as polyarteritis nodosa, can also lead to stroke. A number of coagulopathies can lead to stroke at a young age, including protein C and S deficiencies, factor V-Leiden deficiency, and others. Migraine can lead to persistent motor aura in the Hemiplegic variant, which exists in sporadic and familial forms. Partial epilepsy can lead to postictal paralysis ("Todd's paralysis"), which can also mimic stroke. Mitochondrial encephalomyopathy, lactic acidosis, and stroke-like episodes (MELAS) commonly presents in childhood with stroke syndromes, often accompanied by migraine-like headaches. Cerebral autosomal dominant arteriopathy with subcortical infarcts and leukoencephalopathy (CADASIL) can present (rarely) in the adolescent age group.

Signs and symptoms of stroke are similar in adolescents and adults. This patient probably had an occlusion of a middle cerebral branch (asymmetry of face, arm, and leg symptoms, and relative sparing of sensation). Diagnostic workup should be thorough and include MRI of the head with DWI, MR venography, and MR arteriography in hopes of localizing the pathology. Doppler studies of the cervical vessels can shed light on proximal arterial flow. Echocardiogram is essential in ruling out valvular disease, patient foramen ovale (PFO), and intracardiac thrombus. Sickle cell disease should be ruled out and coagulation profile should be complete, including anticardiolipin antibody, lupus anticoagulant, protein C, protein S, factor V Leiden, fibrinogen, antinuclear antibody, ESR, blood cultures, toxicology screen, urine amino acids, organic acids and homocysteine, lipid panel, basic chemistry panel, blood count, and lactate. Lumbar puncture should probably be done in all young people with stroke to rule out meningeal infection or inflammation.

While this workup is progressing—probably beginning with MRI and MRA, all the basic labs and toxicology screen, and if possible, echocardiography and cervical artery Doppler studies—is there treatment that should be started? Clearly there are some childhood strokes that could benefit from intravenous thrombolysis. The problem, besides the lack of controlled studies of this treatment, is that childhood stroke etiology is more varied than adult stroke, leading to a large number of causes NOT expected to benefit from tissue plasminogen activator (tPA). Is there any other intervention that might help? Good hydration, permissive mild hypertension, and treatment of the underlying mechanism as fast as possible are really the best options. If seizure is suspected, EEG should be done to attempt to confirm, and anticonvulsants can be started if there is strong suspicion. Anticoagulants are rarely used. If intracranial pressure increases, which can happen in particularly large strokes, as in adults, intracranial pressure monitoring can be very helpful in directing measures to reduce pressure, such as diuretics and even hemicranicetomy. This kind of increase in intracranial pressure is fortunately rare in children. Sickle cell disease is managed by repeat blood transfusions.

A stroke can be emotionally devastating to any patient, but especially to children and adolescents. Careful and thorough explanations and appropriate counseling are both highly important.

KEY POINTS TO REMEMBER

- The causes of stroke in childhood and adolescence include those underlying adult stroke, as well as a number of other diseases, including hypercoagulable disorders and vascular anomalies.
- Some conditions can mimic stroke, including hemiplegic migraine and postictal paralysis.

- While tPA is probably a useful treatment in many adolescent strokes, the disparity in causation of childhood/adolescent stroke makes it difficult to design a protocol.
- Anticoagulation is only indicated in the acute treatment of stroke in this age group when there is a clear cardiac thromboembolic source or cerebral venous thrombosis (and is generally standard treatment of arterial dissection as well).

Further Reading

Amlie-Lefond C, Benedict S, Bernard T, et al, and the International Paediatric Stroke Study Investigators: Thrombolysis in children with arterial ischemic stroke: initial results from the International Paediatric Stroke Study. *Stroke*. 2007;38:485.

Arnold M, Steinlin M, Baumann A, et al. Thrombolysis in childhood stroke–report of 2 Cases and review of the literature. *Stroke*. 2009;40: 801-807.

McGlennan C, Ganesan V. Delays in investigation and management of acute arterial ischaemic stroke in children. *Dev Med Child Neurol*. 2008;50:537-540.

Index

A

abbreviations used in text, xiii

abdominal pain, and syncope, 43–44

abuse, detecting and treating, 139–141

acute ataxia in a child, 135–138

acute disseminated encephalomyelitis (ADEM), 136

agitated delirium, 7–11

  sedation of, 8

akathisia, and neuroleptic medications, 58

alcohol intoxication

  and agitated delirium, 9–10, 11

Alzheimer's disease, and cognitive dysfunction, 31

amaurosis fugax, 48

amnesia, following concussion, 145

"analgesic rebound" headache, 86–87

aneurysm

  and acute severe facial pain, 98

  and thunderclap headache, 55

angiotensin converting enzyme level test, in isolated vertigo, 37

ankle-jerk reflex, and lumbar radiculopathy, 90

anticholinergics

  overdose with, 59–60

  and pupillary changes, 8

anticoagulation therapy

  in basilar artery occlusion (BAO), 75

  blood pressure monitoring during, 72

  contraindications *vs.* benefits, 69, 70, 71

  and lumbar puncture, 22, 23

anticonvulsant medication, initiating, 120–123

antidepressants

  overdose with cyclic antidepressants, 59

  and pupillary changes, 8

antiemetic medications, 128

antiepileptic drugs

  and agitated delirium, 10

  in febrile seizure, 133

  initiating treatment with, 120–123

antihistamines, overdose with, 59

antinausea medications, 128, 129

antithrombotic therapy, with oral aspirin, 79

aortic dissection, and syncope, 43–44

arrhythmias

  and intractable status epilepticus, 84

  and syncope, 43

arthritis, and lumbosacral spinal stenosis, 90

ataxia, in a pediatric patient, 135–138

  causes, 136

atherothrombosis, and acute stroke in an adolescent, 148

atypical facial pain, 99–100

B

bacterial meningitis, treatment for, 6

basilar artery occlusion (BAO), 74–75

benign positional vertigo *vs.* vestibular neuronitis, 38

bleeding diathesis, and contraindications to lumbar puncture, 22–23

blood clot "extraction"

  in basilar artery occlusion (BAO), 75

  in treatment for acute stroke, 67

blood pressure

  and focally stenotic artery, 79

  and hyperperfusion syndrome, 15

  monitoring during anticoagulation therapy, 72

  monitoring during intractable status epilepticus, 82

blood pressure *(Cont.)*
  monitoring in basilar artery occlusion
    (BAO), 75
  and syncope, 44
bradycardia, and syncope, 43

C

Call-Fleming syndrome, 54
cardiac monitoring
  in presyncope, 38
  in syncope, 44
cardioembolic stroke, and contraindications
    to anticoagulation, 69–72
cardiovascular disease, and isolated
    vertigo, 39
carotid arterial dissection, and thunderclap
    headache, 55
carotid disease, and intra-arterial
    angiography, 14
carotid endarterectomy, post-surgical
    sequelae, 13–16
carotid sinus syncope, 44
cerebral ischemia, and persistent migraine
    aura, 20
cerebrospinal fluid (CSF)
  in acute ataxia in a child, 136, 137
  in acute monocular vision loss, 50
  in acute stroke in an adolescent, 149
  in agitated delirium, 9
  in bacterial meningitis, 105
  in coma with fever, 4–5
  in diffuse weakness, 27
  in febrile delirium with rigidity, 59
  in febrile seizure, 132–133, 133
  in first seizure, 120, 123
  in isolated vertigo, 36–37, 39
  in meningitis, 5
  in severe intractable headache, 86
  in thunderclap headache, 55, 56
  in trigeminal neuralgia, 98
cerebrovascular disease, and isolated
    vertigo, 39

cervical spinal stenosis, treatment in
    elderly, 31
chest pain, and syncope, 43–44
chest x-ray, in syncope, 43
child abuse
  detecting and treating, 139–141
  types, 140
cluster headaches *vs.* trigeminal neuralgia, 98
coagulation dysfunction, and lumbar
    puncture, 22, 23
coagulation profile, in acute stroke in an
    adolescent, 149
cognitive function
  and Alzheimer's disease, 31
  pre- and postconcussion, 145
  and subcortical ischemic disease, 31
coma with fever, 3–6
combative patients, 7–11
competency, determining in neurological
    patients, 103–106
complete blood count (CBC)
  in acute stroke in an adolescent, 149
  in confusion in childhood, 140
  in febrile delirium with rigidity, 59
  in febrile seizure, 132, 133
  and hypercoagulability, 78
computed tomography (CT)
  in acute ataxia in a child, 136, 137
  in agitated delirium, 9
  in basilar artery occlusion (BAO), 74, 75
  in concussion, 144
  in confused patients, 11, 105
  in febrile delirium with rigidity, 59
  in febrile seizure, 132
  in first seizure, 120, 123
  in intracranial mass lesion, 116–117
  in isolated vertigo, 36
  in nonepileptic spells, 112
  in pediatric patient with migraine,
    127, 128
  in persistent migraine aura, 19
  in presyncope, 38

I

idiopathic thrombocytopenic purpura,
21–24
imbalance, and transient ischemic attack
(TIA), 74
immunosuppressed patients, and
intracranial mass lesions, 116
intra-arterial angiography
in carotid disease, 14
in transient ischemic attack (TIA), 79
intra-arterial stenting, in basilar artery
occlusion (BAO), 75
intra-arterial thrombotic therapy, in
postoperative thrombotic stroke, 14
intracerebral hemorrhage
after concussion, 144, 146
and agitated delirium, 9
and hyperperfusion syndrome, 14–15
intracranial mass lesions
and first seizure, 120
in HIV infection, 115–118
intracranial pressure
and acute stroke in an adolescent, 149
and lumbar puncture, 4
intractable headache, 85–88
intractable status epilepticus, 81–84
intubation, in status epilepticus, 82–83
iritis, 48
ischemia
and acute stroke after 3 hours, 66
ischemia of the retina, 48, 49, 50
in persistent migraine aura, 18
preventing recurrent cerebral ischemia,
71
progressive posterior-circulation
ischemia, 73–76
recurrent transient ischemia, 78

L

labyrinthitis
and acute ataxia in a child, 137
and isolated vertigo, 36

Leber optic neuropathy, 50
legal dilemmas with intransigent patients,
104–105
leukoencephalopathy, 116
ligament strain *vs.* lumbar radiculopathy, 90
lightheadedness
and cardiac evaluation, 39
isolated vertigo, 36, 38
lorazepam, in ethanol withdrawal, 105
low-molecular-weight heparin (LMWH), 71
lumbar puncture
in acute ataxia in a child, 136, 137
in acute monocular vision loss, 50
in acute stroke in an adolescent, 149
in bacterial meningitis, 105
and coagulation dysfunction, 22, 23
complications of, 23
contraindications to, 21–24, 31, 140
in diffuse weakness, 27
in febrile delirium with rigidity, 59
in febrile seizure, 132–133, 133
in first seizure, 120, 123
indications for, 11, 22
and intracranial mass lesions, 117, 118
in isolated vertigo, 36–37, 39
safety of, 4, 7
in severe intractable headache, 86
in thunderclap headache, 55, 56
in trigeminal neuralgia, 98
lumbar radiculopathy, 89–92
lupus, and optic neuropathy, 49
Lyme disease, and facial pain, 98
Lyme titer, in isolated vertigo, 37

M

MacArthur Competence Assessment
Test, 104
magnetic resonance imaging (MRI)
in acute ataxia in a child, 136, 137
in acute stroke in an adolescent, 148
in basilar artery occlusion (BAO), 75
in cardioembolic stroke, 70–71, 72

pulmonary embolism, and syncope, 44
pupillary changes
  after cataract surgery, 38
  in agitated delirium, 8–9
  drug-induced, 8–9
  Marcus Gunn pupil, 47, 48

R

rabies *vs.* other viral encephalitides, 58
radiculopathy, acute lumbar, 89–92
"re-expression," of symptoms from previous
  stroke, 78
reflexes
  and acute ataxia in a child, 135
  and functional paraparesis, 110
  and lumbar radiculopathy, 90
respiratory function, monitoring
  in diffuse weakness, 27
  in intractable status epilepticus, 82
retina, and acute monocular visual loss, 48,
  49, 50
retinal artery and vein occlusion, 49
return-to-play guidelines, after concussion,
  145, 146
reversible cerebral vasoconstriction
  syndrome (RCVS), 54
rigidity, with fever and delirium, 57–61
roseola, and acute ataxia in children, 137

S

sarcoidosis, and acute severe facial pain, 98
schizophrenia, and patients with febrile
  delirium, 57–61
sedation
  of agitated patients, 8, 10, 11
  in intractable status epilepticus, 83
  of intransigent patients, 105
  of pediatric patients with severe migraine,
    129
seizure
  and acute stroke in an adolescent, 149
  etiology of, 120

febrile seizure, 131–134
first seizure, 119–123
  and hyperperfusion syndrome, 14–15
  initiating anticonvulsant medication,
    120–123
  intractable status epilepticus, 81–84
  lifestyle changes to raise seizure threshold,
    122
  medications to treat, 82–83, 84
  nonepileptic spells, 111–114
  potential first-time causes, 121
  and syncope, 44
  and thrombocytopenic purpura, 21
  See also epilepsy
serotonin syndrome (SS)
  presentation of, 60
  vs. neuroleptic malignant syndrome, 58
sexual abuse, and confused pediatric
  patient, 140
sickle-cell disease, and acute stroke in an
  adolescent, 148, 149
simple febrile seizures, features, 132
single-photon emission computed
  tomography (SPECT)
  in hyperperfusion syndrome, 15
  in intracranial mass lesion, 117
skull fractures, after concussion, 144
social work team, and discharge to
  long-term care, 31–32
Solitaire® flow restoration device, in acute
  stroke, 67
somatization, and syncope, 44
somatosensory evoked potentials (SSEP),
  30–31
sphenoid sinusitis, and thunderclap
  headache, 55
spinal cord injury, 93–96
  initial treatment of, 95
  primary *vs.* secondary injury, 94, 95
  syndromes, 94–95
spinal cord lesions
  and acute ataxia in a child, 136

Lightning Source UK Ltd.
Milton Keynes UK
UKOW031902260613

212815UK00010B/37/P